The National Foundation – March of Dimes
Birth Defects: Original Article Series Volume XII, Number 1, 1976

CANCER AND GENETICS

**The 1975 BIRTH DEFECTS CONFERENCE
Held at Kansas City, Missouri
Sponsored by the University of Kansas Medical Center
College of Health Sciences and Hospital
and The National Foundation – March of Dimes**

Editor: **Daniel Bergsma, M.D.,** Vice President for Professional Education, The National Foundation

Associate Editors: **R. Neil Schimke, M.D.,** Departments of Medicine and Pediatrics, University of Kansas Medical Center, Kansas City, Kansas

Robert L. Summitt, M.D., Department of Pediatrics, University of Tennessee, Memphis, Tennessee

David J. Harris, M.D., Department of Pediatrics, Children's Mercy Hospital, Kansas City, Missouri

Assistant Editor: **Natalie Paul,** The National Foundation

ALAN R. LISS, INC., NEW YORK, N. Y.

To enhance medical communication in the birth defects field,
The National Foundation publishes the *Birth Defects Atlas and
Compendium*, an *Original Article Series*, *Syndrome Identification*,
a *Reprint Series* and provides a series of films and related brochures.

Further information can be obtained from:
Professional Education Department
The National Foundation — March of Dimes
1275 Mamaroneck Avenue
White Plains, New York 10605

Published by
Alan R. Liss, Inc.
150 Fifth Avenue
New York, New York 10011

Received for publication October 22, 1975

Library of Congress Cataloging in Publication Data

Birth Defects Conference, Kansas City, Mo., 1975.
    Cancer and genetics.

    (Birth defects original article series; v. 12, no. 1)
    Includes bibliographical references and indexes.
    1. Cancer — Genetic aspects — Congresses. 2. Deformities —
Genetic aspects — Congresses. I. Bergsma, Daniel. II. Kansas.
University. Medical Center. III. National Foundation. IV. Title.
V. Series.
[DNLM: 1. Abnormalities — Congresses. 2. Genetics, Human —
Congresses. 3. Neoplasms — Familial and genetic — Congresses.
4. Neoplasms — Etiology — Congresses. W1 BI966 v. 12 no. 1/
[QZ202 B619b 1975]
RG626.B63 vol. 12, no. 1 [RC262] 616' .043'08s
ISBN 0-8451-1002-0   [616' .043]   75-43622

Printed in U. S. A.

Table of Contents

Contributors

Claus R. Bartram, Institut für Humangenetik, Universitat Hamburg, Germany

Martha S. Berberich, M. D., Pediatric Resident, Oakland Children's Hospital, Oakland, CA 94601

David Bixler, Ph. D., D. D. S., Departments of Oral–facial and Medical Genetics, Indiana University School of Dentistry, Indianapolis, IN 46202

Marylou Buyse, M. D., Carney Hospital, Boston, MA 02124

Colin J. Condron, M. A., M. D., Chairman, Department of Pediatrics, Orange Memorial Hospital, Orlando, FL 32806

P. Michael Conneally, Ph. D., Department of Medical Genetics, University of Indiana Medical Center, Indianapolis, IN 46202

Victor Escobar, D. D. S., Departments of Oral–facial and Medical Genetics, Indiana University School of Dentistry, Indianapolis, IN 46202

Philip J. Fialkow, M. D., Chief, Medical Service, Veterans Administration Hospital, Seattle, WA 98108

Jan M. Friedman, M. D., Senior Fellow, Veterans Administration Hospital, Seattle, WA 98108

Robert J. Gorlin, D. D. S., M. S., Division of Oral Pathology, University of Minnesota School of Dentistry, Health Sciences Unit, Minneapolis, MN 55455

Judith G. Hall, M. D., Director, Medical Genetics, The Children's Orthopedic Hospital and Medical Center and Assistant Professor, Pediatrics and Medicine, University of Washington School of Medicine, Seattle, WA 98105

Juliet Hananian, M. D., Assistant Professor, Department of Pediatrics, University of Miami, Miami, FL 33152

C. Thomas Hartman, M. D., Department of Pediatrics, Los Angeles County– University of Southern California Medical Center, Los Angeles, CA 90033

Jürgen Herrmann, M. D., Assistant Professor, Pediatrics, Clinical Genetics Center, University of Wisconsin Medical School, Madison, WI 53706

Kurt Hirschhorn, M. D., Division of Medical Genetics, Mount Sinai School of Medicine, New York, NY 10029

William A. Horton, M. D., Epidemiology Branch, NINDS, National Institutes of Health, Bethesda, MD 20014

Charles E. Jackson, M. D., Chief, Genetics Section, Department of Medicine, Henry Ford Hospital, Detroit, MI 48202

Charles H. Kirkpatrick, M. D., Head, Clinical Allergy and Hypersensitivity Section, LCI, National Institute of Allergy and Infectious Diseases, National Institutes of Health, Bethesda, MD 20014

Kjell Koch, M. D., Associate Professor, Department of Pediatrics, University of Miami, Miami, FL 33152

Robert W. Miller, M. D., Epidemiology Branch, National Cancer Institute, National Institutes of Health, Bethesda, MD 20014

John J. Mulvihill, M. D., Head, Clinical Genetics Section, Epidemiology Branch, National Cancer Institute, National Institutes of Health, Bethesda, MD 20014

Eberhard Passarge, M. D., Head, Division of Cytogenetics and Clinical Genetics, Universitat Hamburg, Institut für Humangenetik, Universitats-Krankenhaus Eppendorf, Germany

Guy Photopulos, M. D., Division of Oncology, Department of Obstetrics and Gynecology, The University of North Carolina School of Medicine, Chapel Hill, NC 27514

Vincent M. Riccardi, M. D., Genetics Unit, University of Colorado Medical Center, Denver, CO 80220

Joe Leigh Simpson, M. D., Associate Professor of Obstetrics and Gynecology, Prentice Women's Hospital and Maternity Center, Northwestern University School of Medicine, Chicago, IL 60611

Glen W. Sizemore, M. D., Endocrinology Department, Mayo Clinic, Rochester, MN 55901

Michael Swift, M. D., Chief, Division of Medical Genetics, Biological Sciences Research Center, University of North Carolina, Chapel Hill, NC 27514

Armen H. Tashjian, Jr., M. D., Pharmacology Department, Harvard School of Dental Medicine, Harvard Medical School, Boston, MA 02115

Miriam G. Wilson, M. D., Department of Pediatrics, Los Angeles County–University of Southern California Medical Center, Los Angeles, CA 90033

Peculiarities in the Distribution of Cancer as Clues to Its Origins: Host Factors

Robert W. Miller, MD

Important clues to the origins of cancer come from study of peculiarities in its distribution. In such studies, the purer the diagnosis, the greater the opportunity for developing new insight. An obvious first step in purifying the diagnosis of cancer is to classify it by histologic type, rather than simply by anatomic site.

Peculiarities in the distribution of cancer by histologic type may be found with regard to host factors (eg age, sex, race, family or preexistent disease) or environmental factors, (eg geography, occupation, drugs or habits). Study of host factors defines who is most, or least susceptible to specific neoplasms. One can then consider why these marked excesses or deficiencies occur, and in so doing may determine something new about the fundamental biology of cancer. Such information may be obtained from observational studies of man, and not from laboratory studies on animals, as, for example, the relation of Down syndrome to leukemia.[1] Further elaboration of the significance of such findings may depend heavily on laboratory research.

Some important findings lie very close to the surface, but go undiscovered because that kind of research-probing has not been fashionable. In the epidemiology of cancer, attention still tends to be focused on the most frequent neoplasms (because of their public health importance) rather than on rare cancers which may reveal carcinogenic processes applicable far beyond the specific neoplasm itself. Much of the first half of this volume is based on information drawn from non-mainstream studies in the past decade.

PECULIARITIES IN DISTRIBUTION BY AGE, SEX, AND RACE

Dynamic changes in mortality by single year of age may be seen in specific

Birth Defects: Original Article Series, Volume XII, Number 1, pages 1–5

forms of childhood cancer. Among U.S. white children there are marked peaks in mortality from 8 neoplasms within the first 5 years of life (acute lymphocytic leukemia, neuroblastoma, Wilms tumor, retinoblastoma, sacrococcygeal teratoma, rhabdomyosarcoma, ependymoma and hepatoblastoma).[2] This early age of occurrence indicates that the influences responsible are largely prenatal. The patterns for other childhood cancers are quite different. Acute myelogenous leukemia has a constant mortality rate throughout childhood, except for a small peak in adolescence.[3] The patterns for the 3 main forms of lymphoma differ from one another and from leukemia.[2] Death rates from lymphosarcoma rise steeply in frequency at about 2 years of age in boys and reach a plateau that continues throughout the pediatric years. The picture is quite different for girls, who have only one-third the rates that boys do — a very large sex difference. Hodgkin disease shows an upturn in rates in about mid-childhood (suggesting an age-related fault in immunologic development[4]), whereas reticulum cell sarcoma increases progressively with age. The 2 main forms of bone cancer, osteosarcoma and Ewing tumor, have similar patterns in U.S. white children, but remarkably, Ewing tumor is almost absent in U.S. blacks[2] and among blacks in Africa.[5] U.S. blacks also fail to show the peak at 4 years of age in mortality from acute lymphocytic leukemia that is seen in U.S. whites.[6] These racial differences suggest a genetic basis for resistance to certain forms of cancer.

INTERNATIONAL DIFFERENCES

Under the sponsorship of the International Union Against Cancer, a world-wide survey was conducted by mail to determine the relative frequencies of type-specific childhood neoplasms in major pediatric centers throughout the world. Data were collected on more than 40,000 children with cancer. Among the interesting findings were the following. The high frequency of pinealoma among the Japanese was confirmed.[7] There was a marked excess of skin cancer in the genetic disorder xeroderma pigmentosum throughout North Africa. This finding, well-known to the physicians of the area[8] had not previously been brought to international attention.

As has been noticed by others, the frequency of Wilms tumor appeared to be the most constant of all childhood neoplasms throughout the world.[9] In consequence, when use is made of hospital data and the population-at-risk cannot be defined, Wilms tumor may be used as a yardstick against which the frequencies of other childhood tumors can be measured; that is, a ratio can be created in which Wilms tumor is used as the denominator and the number of cancers of another type are used as the numerator. When neuroblastoma was studied in this way, a gradual decline in the ratio was observed in Europe, from west to east, and the opposite effect was observed with regard to Hodgkin disease (R. W. Miller, unpublished data). The lowest rates for neuroblastoma occurred in black Africa, in contrast to the lack of difference between the rates for the U.S. blacks and U.S. whites. The progressive change in rates for neuroblastoma and Hodgkin disease across Europe, and the possible migrant effect in blacks, suggest an environmental agent as a determinant in the occurrence of these tumors.

FAMILIAL CANCER AND MULTIPLE PRIMARY CANCERS

Apart from the known genetically determined cancers, certain other neoplasms seem to aggregate excessively in families. These cancers may be of a single histologic type, as in a Boston family in which 7, and possibly 10 members had ovarian carcinoma,[10] or may be of specific dissimilar cell types, the rarity of which makes their occurrence in several unrelated families seem unlikely to be due to chance. Soft-tissue tumors in sibs during childhood have been found in multiple families in which other cancers, especially of the breast in young females, affect close relatives.[11,12] Glioma, adrenal cortical carcinoma and osteosarcoma — seemingly unrelated histologic types, have been observed in first-degree relatives in several families.[13] Thus, it appears that the same cancers that occur as double primaries may also be distributed excessively in families.

Similarly the elements of syndromes involving cancer and noncancerous disease may also be spread through the family rather than concentrated in one individual, as for example in an American Indian family studied by my colleagues,[14] in which 3 members had osteosarcoma, one had synostosis of the radius and ulna, and several had erythrocytic macrocytosis. When cancers aggregate excessively in families with or without other disorders, there is an opportunity for extensive laboratory investigation to determine if subclinical features in common can be found in members with various manifestations of disease as well as those who are phenotypically normal.

CANCER AND CONGENITAL MALFORMATIONS

In the mid-1950s, several reports appeared confirming an observation apparently long known to clinicians that there was an association between Down syndrome and leukemia. These observations, coupled with others of similar nature, led to the realization that chromosomal abnormalities may be present in groups at high risk of leukemia.[15] With the development of banding techniques for cytogenetic study, it has become increasingly apparent that this feature of high-risk groups also applies to leukemia in general, at least of the myelogenous type.[16,17]

About 10 years after the first reports of the occurrence of the Down syndrome with leukemia, it was found that inborn immunodeficiency states predispose to lymphoma.[18] Subsequently it was found that the impairment had to be at least in part cell-mediated.[19] Thus, a marked difference was drawn between the primary mechanisms apparently involved in leukemogenesis as compared with genesis of lymphoma.

At about the same time, by simply abstracting information from 440 hospital records of children with Wilms tumor, it was found that sporadic congenital aniridia was associated with this neoplasm.[20] In addition, the tumor also occurred excessively in patients with various manifestations of growth excess: congenital hemihypertrophy, hamartomas or the visceral cytomegaly (Beckwith-Wiedemann) syndrome.[21] These and later observations led to the conclusion that factors producing various manifestations of growth excess, at times involving anatomically unrelated portions of the body, have something to do with the genesis of nephroblastoma. Although certain of the malformations that predispose to Wilms tumor have no known connection with one another (eg aniridia and hemihypertrophy), each has a feature in common with the others, namely, renal malformation. Thus, it appears that certain anomalies of the kidney, occurring alone or as part of a syndrome, give rise to Wilms tumor. By contrast, neuroblastoma, which seems to have prenatal determinants, as reflected by its peak occurrence soon after birth, has no strong association with any form of congenital anomaly. Thus, it is clear that each of these childhood tumors, leukemia, lymphoma, Wilms tumor and neuroblastoma involve dissimilar mechanisms in their genesis. From these rarities of nature new understanding of the cancerous process has been derived. These observations made largely at the bedside have given new directions to laboratory research in exploring the neoplastic process.

REFERENCES

1. Miller, R. W.: Neoplasia and Down's syndrome. Ann. N.Y. Acad. Sci. 171:637–644, 1970.
2. Miller, R. W. and Dalager, N. A.: U.S. childhood cancer deaths by cell type 1960–68. J. Pediatr. 85:664–668, 1974.
3. Court Brown, W. M. and Doll, R.: Leukemia in childhood and young adult life. Trends in mortality in relation to aetiology. Br. Med. J. 1:981–988, 1961.
4. Miller, R. W.: Mortality in childhood Hodgkin's disease. JAMA 198:1216–1217, 1966.
5. Davies, J. N. P.: Childhood tumors. In Templeton (ed.) Tumours in a Tropical Country. New York: Springer-Verlag, 1973, pp. 306–343.
6. Miller, R. W.: Environmental agents in cancer. Yale J. Biol. Med. 37:487–507, 1965.
7. Araki, C. and Matsumoto, S.: Statistical reevaluation of pinealoma and related tumors in Japan. J. Neurosurg. 30:146, 1969.
8. Marshall, J.: Skin Diseases in Africa. Capetown: Maske W. Miller, Ltd., 1964, p. 91.
9. Editorial: An index reference cancer. Lancet 2:651, 1973.
10. Li, F. P., Fraumeni, J. F., Jr. and Dalager, N. A.: Ovarian cancers in the young: Epidemiologic observations. Cancer 32:969–972, 1973.
11. Li, F. P. and Fraumeni, J. F., Jr.: Soft-tissue sarcomas, breast cancer and other neoplasms. A familial syndrome. Ann. Intern. Med. 71:747–752, 1969.

12. Li, F. P. and Fraumeni, J. F., Jr: Rhabdomyosarcoma in children: Epidemiologic study and identification of a familial cancer syndrome. J. Natl. Cancer Inst. 43:1365–1373, 1969.
13. Miller, R. W.: Deaths from childhood leukemia and solid tumors among twins and other sibs in the United States, 1960–67. J. Natl. Cancer Inst. 46:203–209, 1971.
14. Mulvihill, J. J.: Unpublished observations.
15. Miller, R. W.: Persons at exceptionally high risk of leukemia. Cancer Res. 27:2420–2423, 1967.
16. Miller, R. W.: Features in common of persons at high risk of leukemia. In The Biology of Radiation Carcinogenesis. New York: Raven Press. (In press.)
17. Levan, G. and Mitelman, F.: Clustering of aberrations to specific chromosomes in human neoplasms. Hereditas 79:156–160, 1975.
18. Peterson, R. D. A., Cooper, M. D. and Good, R. A.: Disorders of the thymus and other lymphoid tissues. Prog. Med. Genet. 4:1–31, 1965.
19. Waldmann, T. A., Strober, W. and Blaese, R. M.: Immunodeficiency disease and malignancy. Various immunologic deficiencies of man and the role of immune processes in the control of malignant disease. Ann. Intern. Med. 77:605–628, 1972.
20. Miller, R. W., Fraumeni, J. F., Jr. and Manning, M. D.: Association of Wilms' tumor with aniridia and hemihypertrophy and other congenital malformations. N. Engl. J. Med. 270:922–927, 1964.
21. Miller, R. W.: Etiology of childhood cancer. In Sutow, W. W., Vietti, T. J. and Fernbach, D. J. (eds.) Clinical Pediatric Oncology, St. Louis: C. V. Mosby, 1973, pp. 7–18.

Some Soft Tissue Heritable Tumors *

Robert J. Gorlin, DDS, MS

When I was asked to present a paper at this conference on soft tissue tumors,
I accepted hesitantly not because I have any flagging interest in the field but because I was not certain that I had sufficient expertise. After brief reflection, I
realized that considerable personal benefit would be gained by review of the
field. At first blush, what appeared to be a well-limned region of knowledge
burgeoned into a plethora of conditions concerning many of which I had but
passing acquaintance and, for some disorders, none at all. One can only select
a few of the myriad conditions that might be discussed. I have chosen a few that
have captured my interest and I hope to make a few more than nugatory remarks
concerning some of them.

MULTIPLE HAMARTOMA AND NEOPLASIA SYNDROME
(COWDEN SYNDROME)

This syndrome was first described by Lloyd and Dennis.[1] Weary et al
published 5 examples of the syndrome, emphasizing its hamartomatous
character and suggesting that it principally involved the skin, GI tract, breasts,
and thyroid.[2] Gentry et al reported additional cases.[3,4]

The syndrome is inherited as an autosomal dominant trait.[3] Fibroadenoma-
tosis, virginal hypertrophy, and carcinoma of the breast have been described.
Thyroid alterations have included fetal adenoma, follicular adenocarcinoma
and goiter.

A wide variety of other neoplasms or hamartomas have been noted: ovarian
cysts, meningioma of the ear canal, angiomatous lesions of soft and hard tissues
and lipomas, both subcutaneous and retroperitoneal. Angiomyomas have been

*This study was made possible by USPHS Program Grant in Oral Pathology DE 1770.

Birth Defects: Original Article Series, Volume XII, Number 1, **pages 7—14**
© **1976 The National Foundation**

described in the limbs. Colonic polyps of various types are found: ganglio-neuromatous, retention, hyperplastic, adenomatous, and rarely adenocarcinomatous changes in adenomatous polyps.

The pinnas, lateral neck, nasal, periorbital, glabellar, perioral areas and dorsum of hands and forearms are the most frequently involved sites of lichenoid and papillomatous lesions. Histologic examinations suggest that they are hamartomas of hair follicle origin similar to inverted follicular keratoses. The palms may exhibit waxy punctate keratoderma.[5] Hydronephrosis has been described. However, in one case it was thought to be secondary to a huge retroperitoneal lipoma.[6]

Papular lesions of the lips and gingiva and, to a lesser extent, the palate, as well as papillomatous lesions of the buccal, faucial, and oropharyngeal mucosa have been noted in most patients.[7] The tongue is pebbly and fissured.

MULTIPLE CHEMODECTOMAS

Carotid body tumors or chemodectomas may be observed at any age, but there is a predilection for middle-aged individuals. They are usually sporadic and unilateral. When bilateral, they are often (about 35%) familial. Sporadic cases are rarely (3%) bilateral.

Chase apparently first noted familial occurrence.[8] He reported 2 sisters, one with bilateral carotid body tumors, the other with a unilateral tumor. Since then, numerous cases of these tumors in 2 or more generations have been reported. Autosomal dominant inheritance is clearly indicated.

Of noteworthy mention is the report of Chedid and Jao,[9] who found associated chronic obstructive lung disease in 3 of 4 affected sibs. This raises several interesting questions, some direct, others tangential, none of which will be answered here, but nevertheless merit our consideration regarding the basis for the genetic proclivity of the bilateral tumor.

First, tangentially — hereditary pulmonary emphysema is linked with $alpha_1$-antitrypsin deficiency. Homozygotes nearly always develop chronic obstructive lung disease by 50 years of age. Heterozygotes have a more benign disorder potentiated by cigarette smoking.

More directly, the carotid body as a chemoreceptor organ responds to changes in pO_2, pCO_2, and pH. Bilateral enlargement of the carotid bodies was found in Quechua Indians living in the Peruvian Andes, in contrast to those living at sea level — presumably a physiologic response to hypoxia. Additional weight is given to this argument based on carotid body weight in patients with cor pulmonale, Pickwickian syndrome, and emphysema.[10,11] Hyperplastic carotid bodies are found in animals living at high altitudes.[12] Furthermore, the frequency of carotid body tumors is 10 times as great in individuals living at high altitudes compared with those living at sea level.[13]

In essence, this evidence raises the question whether chemodectomas are not true neoplasms but only hyperplasias produced by increased demand on the chemoreceptive and/or neuroendocrine functions in genetically susceptible individuals. Investigation of this puzzle is bound to yield answers.

BLUE RUBBER BLEB NEVUS

Bean defined the blue rubber bleb nevus syndrome as multiple vascular, 1–20 mm, nipple- or bladder-like lesions of the skin, especially of the trunk and upper arms, and mucous membranes, which may be accompanied by gastrointestinal bleeding and hepatic and pulmonary angiomas.[14,15] Medulloblastoma of the cerebellum has also been noted.[16] In some cases, the lesions are painful and sweat.

In several families the disorder has exhibited autosomal dominant inheritance.[17–20] Oral angiomas have been found in several cases.

Microscopically, there are large numbers of dilated vascular spaces whose walls are often thrown into folds. The vascular spaces are separated by smooth muscle or fibrous connective tissue.[18]

MULTIPLE SEBACEOUS ADENOMAS AND GASTROINTESTINAL CARCINOMA

The association of multiple sebaceous adenomas and gastrointestinal carcinoma has recently been described.[21–23] Several cases have been reported.[24–28] The cancer tends to arise in the colon and apparently has low-grade malignancy.

Multiple sebaceous tumors most often involve the trunk, head and neck, and develop after the visceral carcinoma is diagnosed. Epidermal skin tumors (squamous cell carcinoma, keratoacanthoma, benign keratosis, verruca) are apparently part of the syndrome.[27]

Among 11 cases, a family history of colonic cancer was present in 5 and breast cancer in 2 individuals. The father of 3 patients had adenocarcinoma of the colon but mention of the presence of multiple sebaceous adenomas and other skin tumors was made only by Jakobiec.[27]

Autosomal dominant inheritance is possible but assignment to that category is premature.

LIPOMATOSIS

We will consider 2 different conditions: multiple lipomatosis and symmetric lipomatosis (Launois-Bensaude syndrome).

Multiple lipomatosis is certainly inherited as an autosomal dominant trait.[29–37] The tumors tend to be symmetric, soft, and usually first appear in the third to fifth decades. Usually painless, they may be associated with pain. They are often scattered over the upper limbs, trunk and neck and vary in size from a few cm to as great as 25 cm in diameter. From a few to hundreds may be present. Elevated serum cholesterol has been found in a few cases.[34,38]

The second disorder, symmetric lipomatosis, is known as Fetthals, Madelung disease, or Launois-Bensaude syndrome. The term Fetthals is a poor one since the nonencapsulated, firm, nonpainful fat deposits, while often involving the neck, may be symmetrically distributed to the submental, pre- and postauricular, supraclavicular, paravertebral in the upper back, axillas, groin, etc. This is probably a genetic heterogeneity. One syndrome which seems to be emerging has been called "familial cervical lipodysplasia" which, in my opinion, is not well-named, since it involves fat deposits around the neck, shoulders, buffalo hump area, and groin. The limbs are lean. Phlebectasia, varices, or coronary heart disease has been found in several members as well as insulin resistance, hyperglycemia, cirrhosis, hyperuricemia and/or gouty arthritis, and type IV lipoproteinemia. Inheritance is autosomal dominant.[39-49] Not all of these patients have manifested all the above signs or symptoms, or at least their presence was not documented. Possibly the patient by Kurzweg and Spencer is an additional example.[38] Telangiectasia was noted.

Kadish et al[49] found failure of free fatty acids to rise to expected levels during fasting and after glucose administration — in effect, a functional sympathetic denervation. They further noted that the fatty deposits are similar to those of brown fat.

MULTIPLE CUTANEOUS ANGIOLIPOMAS

Multiple cutaneous angiolipomas usually develop after puberty and are manifested as tender, subcutaneous nodules of the trunk and limbs. They do not occur on the face, scalp, palms or soles. They are encapsulated and contain varying proportions of adipose and vascular tissues. Many hundreds of lesions may be present.[50] One must differentiate this lesion from the rather rare infiltrating angiolipoma which has the capability of invading bone, muscle, nerve or fibrous connective tissue and requires wide excision for removal.[51]

Clinical, pharmacologic and pathologic studies have not revealed the cause of the pain.[52]

Autosomal dominant inheritance of multiple cutaneous angiolipomas is possible. They have been demonstrated in at least 2 generations.[52,53] The infiltratory angiolipoma has no familial predilection.[51]

CUTANEOUS LEIOMYOMATA

Multiple cutaneous leiomyomata of pilar origin manifest autosomal dominant inheritance with incomplete penetrance. Our personal experience is limited to seeing a single kindred of 3 affected generations. While the literature is not inundated with case reports, the evidence seems to support this contention. Affected sibs with normal parents have been noted.[54–57] However, all members of the families were not examined. Concordant identical twins have been reported, which proves nothing.[58,59] Early familial cases were reviewed by Kloepfer et al[54] and Koryn-Heydt.[60]

The lesions usually appear around the age of 20 years on the trunk, arms, or face. There may be only a few or literally hundreds. They are firm, often grouped, and range in size from 1–15 mm in diameter. They are usually skin colored to reddish brown, mobile but fixed to underlying tissues, tender to slight pressure but exquisitely painful to sudden changes in the ambient temperature or on injection of adrenaline.

Microscopically, they are easily identified. The leiomyoma is separated from the normal epithelium by a thin layer of normal connective tissue but is not encapsulated. Elegant demonstration may be effected by means of van Gieson, Masson trichrome, or reticulum stains.

Of considerable importance is the association of uterine leiomyomata (fibroids) or even leiomyosarcoma.[55,59,61–64] The association does not appear to be aleatory.

GLOMANGIOMA

Multiple glomus tumors are inherited as an autosomal dominant trait having been seen in several generations and with male-to-male transmission but there is incomplete penetrance.[65–71] Sibs with normal parents have also been reported.[72,73]

The bluish to reddish masses measuring 0.1–4 cm which resemble cavernous hemangiomas, both clinically and (to the uninitiated) microscopically, may be congenital or may appear within the first 2 decades of life. Some individuals have over 50 separate lesions. They may be asymptomatic, tender to palpation, or remarkably painful even to light touch. They are not usually completely compressible. Some are sensitive to an increase in ambient temperature. Although they are more commonly found on the limbs, they may be generalized over the trunk, and increase in size for a limited time period.

Microscopically, the multiple glomus tumor is unencapsulated and located in the deep corium or fat. It is composed of large, wide, irregularly shaped blood-filled cavities, resembling a cavernous hemangioma. Surrounding the endothelial lining is a 2 to 3-cell thick layer of small polygonal cells with pale cytoplasm and homogeneous round nuclei. In contrast, the solitary glomus tumor (nonhereditary) often appears in individuals over 30 years of age and about 25% are subungual in location. They are often more painful than multiple glomus tumors. Other painful skin tumors include eccrine spiradenoma, angiolipoma, leiomyoma, traumatic neuroma, and blue rubber bleb nevus.

12 / Gorlin

REFERENCES

1. Lloyd, K. M. and Dennis, M.: Cowden's disease. A possible new symptom complex with multiple system involvement. Ann. Intern. Med. 58:136–142, 1963.
2. Weary, P. E., Gorlin, R. J., Gentry, W. C. et al: The multiple hamartoma syndrome (Cowden's disease). Arch. Dermatol. 106:682–690, 1972.
3. Gentry, W. C., Eskritt, N. R. and Gorlin, R. J.: Multiple hamartoma syndrome (Cowden's disease). Arch. Dermatol. 109:521–529, 1974.
4. Gentry, W. C. et al: Cowden syndrome. In Bergsma, D. (ed.): Genetic Forms of Hypogonadism, Birth Defects: Orig. Art. Ser., vol. XI, no. 4. Miami: Symposia Specialists for The National Foundation–March of Dimes, 1975, pp. 137–141.
5. Rosenbluth, M.: Multiple noduli cutanei. An unusual case of multiple noduli cutanei with gingival manifestations. Periodontics 1:81–83, 1963.
6. Lattes, R.: Personal communication, 1974.
7. Carlier, G., Larere, L., Carlier, C. and Houcke, M.: Sclerose tubereuse de Bourneville avec papillomatose de la muqueuse buccale. Rev. Stomatol. Chir. Maxillofac. 72: 607–614, 1971.
8. Chase, W. H.: Familial and bilateral tumours of the carotid body. J. Pathol. Bacteriol. 36:1–12, 1933.
9. Chedid, A. and Jao, W.: Hereditary tumors of the carotid bodies and chronic obstructive pulmonary disease. Cancer 33:1635–1641, 1974.
10. Heath, D., Edwards, C. and Hanes, P.: Postmortem size and structure of the human carotid body. Thorax 25:129–133, 1970.
11. Edwards, C., Heath, D. and Hanes, P.: The carotid body in emphysema and left ventricular hypertrophy. J. Pathol. 104:1–7, 1971.
12. Edwards, C., Heath, D., Hanes, P. et al: The carotid body in animals at high altitude. J. Pathol. 104:231–238, 1970.
13. Saldana, M. J., Salem, L. E. and Travezan, R.: High altitude hypoxia and chemodectomas. Hum. Pathol. 4:251–263, 1973.
14. Bean, W. B.: Vascular Spiders and Related Lesions of the Skin. Springfield: Charles C Thomas, 1958.
15. Bean, W. B.: Rare Diseases and Lesions. Springfield: Charles C Thomas, 1967.
16. Rice, J. S. and Fischer, D. S.: Blue rubber bleb nevus syndrome. Arch. Dermatol. 86:503–511, 1962.
17. Berlyne, G. M. and Berlyne, N.: Anemia due to "blue-rubber bleb" naevus disease. Lancet 2:1275–1277, 1960.
18. Fine, R. M., Derbes, V. J. and Clark, W. H.: Blue rubber bleb nevus. Arch. Dermatol. 84:802–805, 1961.
19. Walshe, M. M., Evans, C. D. and Waren, R. P.: Blue rubber bleb nevus. Br. Med. J. 2: 931–932, 1966.
20. Talbot, S. and Wyatt, E. H.: Blue rubber bleb naevi. Br. J. Dermatol. 82:37–39, 1970.
21. Muir, E. G., Bell, A. J. and Barlow, K. A.: Multiple primary carcinomata of the colon, duodenum and larynx associated with keratoacanthomata of the face. Br. J. Surg. 54: 191–195, 1967.
22. Torre, D.: Multiple sebaceous tumors. Arch. Dermatol. 98:549–552, 1968.
23. Bakker, P. M. and Tjon A Joe, S. S.: Multiple sebaceous gland tumors with multiple tumors of intestinal organs. A new syndrome? Dermatologica 142:50–57, 1971.
24. Rulon, D. B. and Helwig, E. B.: Multiple sebaceous neoplasms of the skin: An association with multiple visceral carcinoma, especially of the colon. Am. J. Clin. Pathol. 60:745–752, 1973.

25. Sciallis, G. F. and Winkelmann, R. K.: Multiple sebaceous adenomas and gastrointestinal carcinoma. Arch. Dermatol. 110:913–916, 1974.
26. Leonard, D. D. and Deaton, W. G.: Multiple sebaceous gland tumors and visceral carcinomas. Arch. Dermatol. 110:917–920, 1974.
27. Jakobiec, F. A.: Sebaceous adenoma of the eyelid and visceral malignancy. Am. J. Ophthalmol. 78:952–960, 1974.
28. Bitran, J. and Pellettiere, E.: Multiple sebaceous gland tumors and internal carcinoma. Torre's syndrome. Cancer 33:835–836, 1974.
29. Siemens, H. W.: Vererbungspathologie. In Jadassohn, J. (ed.): Handbuch der Haut-und Geschlechtskrankheiten. Berlin: Springer, 1929, vol. III.
30. Rauschkolb, J. E.: Multiple lipomatosis. Arch. Dermatol. Syph. 23:160, 1931.
31. Dietel, F.: Handbuch der Haut-und Geschlechtskrankheiten. Jadassohn, J. (ed.): Berlin: Springer, 1932, vol. XII(2).
32. Hillier, F. F.: Hereditary multiple lipomata. Lancet 1:204–205, 1935.
33. Miller, J. K.: Multiple symmetrical lipomatosis. JAMA 106:2059–2060, 1936.
34. Humphrey, A. A. and Kingsley, P. C.: Familial multiple lipomas. Arch. Dermatol. Syph. 37:30–34, 1938.
35. Muller, R.: Observation sur la transmission héréditaire de la lipomatose circonscrite multiple. Dermatologica 103:258–265, 1951.
36. Shanks, J. A., Parenchych, W. and Tuba, J.: Familial multiple lipomatosis. Can. Med. Assoc. J. 77:881–884, 1957.
37. Stephens, F. E. and Isaacson, A.: Hereditary mulitple lipomatosis. J. Hered. 50:51–53, 1959.
38. Kurzweg, F. T. and Spencer, R.: Familial multiple lipomatosis. Am. J. Surg. 82:762–765, 1951.
39. Lyon, I. P.: Adiposis and lipomatosis. Arch. Intern. Med. 6:28–120, 1910.
40. Günther, H.: Klinische Beobachtungen über Lipomatose. Z. Menschl. Vererb-U. Konstit.-Lehre. 5:268–292, 1920.
41. Löwenstein, W.: Über symmetrische, multiple Lipomatosis. Klin. Wochenschr. 8:1614–1618, 1929.
42. Michon, P. and Rose, F.: Adenolipomatose symmétrique familiale. Bull. Soc. Fr. Dermatol. Syph. 42:1005–1007, 1935.
43. Taylor, L. M., Beahrs, O. H. and Fontana, R. S.: Benign symmetric lipomatosis. Mayo Clin. Proc. 36:96–101, 1961.
44. McKusick, V. A.: Medical genetics, 1961. J. Chronic. Dis. 15:417–572, 1962.
45. Strange, D. A. and Fessel, W. J.: Benign symmetrical lipomatosis. JAMA 204:339–340, 1968.
46. Greene, M. L., Glueck, C. J., Fujimoto, W. Y. and Seegmiller, J. E.: Benign symmetrical lipomatosis (Launois-Bensaude adenolipomatosis), with gout and hyperlipoproteinemia. Am. J. Med. 48:239–246, 1970.
47. Ozer, F. L., Lichenstein, J. R., Kwiterovich, P. O. and McKusick, V. A.: A "new" genetic variety of "lipodystrophy." Clin. Res. 21:533, 1973.
48. Nödl, F.: Lipomatose. Dtsch. Med. Wochenschr. 99:1427, 1974.
49. Kadish, M. E., Alsever, R. N. and Block, M. B.: Benign symmetrical lipomatosis. Functional sympathetic denervation of adipose tissue and possible hypertrophy of brown fat. Metabolism 23:937–945, 1974.
50. Howard, W. R. and Helwig, E. B.: Angiolipoma. Arch. Dermatol. 82:924–931, 1960.
51. Lin, J. J. and Lin, F.: Two entities in angiolipoma. A study of 459 cases of lipoma with review of literature on infiltrating angiolipoma. Cancer 34:720–727, 1974.

52. Belcher, R. W., Czarnetski, B. M., Carney, J. F. and Gardner, E.: Multiple (subcutaneous) angiolipomas. Arch. Dermatol. 110:583–585, 1974.

53. Klem, K. K.: Multiple lipoma-angiolipoma. Acta Chir. Scand. 97:527–532, 1949.

54. Kloepfer, H. W., Krafchuk, J., Derbes, V. and Burks, J.: Hereditary multiple leiomyomas of skin. Am. J. Hum. Genet. 10:48–52, 1958.

55. Knoth, W. and Knoth-Born, R. C.: Familiäre uterocutane Leiomyomatose. Z. Haut. Geschlechtskr. 37:191–206, 1964.

56. Nair, B. K. H.: Familial cutaneous leiomyoma. Indian J. Pathol. Bacteriol. 16:75–77, 1973.

57. Verma, K. C., Chawdhry, S. D. and Rathi, K. S.: Cutaneous leiomyomata in two brothers. Br. J. Dermatol. 89:351–353, 1973.

58. Fischer, W. C. and Helwig, E. B.: Leiomyomas of the skin. Arch. Dermatol. 88: 510–520, 1963.

59. Rudner, E. J., Schwartz, O. P. and Grekin, J. N.: Multiple cutaneous leiomyoma in identical twins. Arch. Dermatol. 90:81–82, 1964.

60. Koryn-Heydt, G. E.: Erblich Aplasien, Hyperplasien und Tumoren. In Jadassohn, J. (ed.): Hanbuch der Haut-und Geschlechtskrankheiten. Berlin: Springer, 1966, pp. 585–587.

61. Piredda, A.: Leiomioma cutaneo e fibromiomatosi uterina. Arch. Ital. Derm. 29: 68–75, 1957.

62. Mezzadra, G.: Leiomyoma cutaneo multiple ereditario. Minerva Derm. 40:388–393, 1965.

63. Thomine, E. and Anzani, C.: Métastase cutanée d'un léiomyome utérine. Bull. Soc. Fr. Derm. Syph. 74:170–172, 1967.

64. Reed, W. B., Walker, R. and Horowitz, R.: Cutaneous leiomyomata with uterine leiomyomata. Acta Derm. Venereol. (Stockh.) 53:409–416, 1973.

65. Kaufman, L. R. and Clark, W. T.: Glomus tumors: Report of four cases in the same family. Ann. Surg. 114:1102–1105, 1941.

66. Gorlin, R. J., Fusaro, R. M. and Benton, J. W.: Multiple glomus tumor of the pseudocavernous hemangioma type. Arch. Dermatol. 82:776–778, 1960.

67. Chasseuil, R. and Gautard, J.: Tumeurs glomiques familiales: 6 cas en 4 generations. Bull. Soc. Fr. Dermatol. Syph. 68:635–636, 1961.

68. Nödl, F.: Multiple systematisierte Glomustumoren. Arch. Klin. Exp. Dermatol. 217:405–416, 1963.

69. Schnyder, U. W.: Über Glomustumoren. Dermatologica 131:83–88, 1965.

70. Conant, M. A. and Wiesenfeld, S. L.: Multiple glomus tumors of the skin. Arch. Dermatol. 103:481–485, 1971.

71. Hollins, P. J.: Multiple glomus tumours. Proc. R. Soc. Med. 64:806, 1971.

72. Hueston, J. T.: Multiple painless glomus tumours. Br. Med. J. 1:1212, 1961.

73. Burford, C.: Multiple glomus tumors. Australas. J. Dermatol. 15:35, 1974.

The Relationship of Neoplasia to Disorders of Abnormal Sexual Differentiation

Joe Leigh Simpson, MD and Guy Photopulos, MD

INTRODUCTION

Some disorders of abnormal sexual differentiation are associated with neoplasia more often than expected by probability. This phenomenon is not well understood, although it is not surprising because 1) the relationship between neoplasia and maldevelopment of any organ system is poorly understood, and 2) a satisfactory delineation for most disorders of abnormal sexual differentiation has only recently been possible.

The purpose of this communication is to survey the disorders of abnormal sexual differentiation with respect to frequency of neoplasia. We will 1) summarize the ovarian and testicular tumors that are most commonly associated with disorders of abnormal sexual differentiation; 2) discuss the relationship between cryptorchidism and testicular neoplasia; 3) estimate the risk of neoplasia in various disorders, and 4) suggest clinical management when appropriate, or consider the role of various factors in neoplastic transformation.

CLINICAL DELINEATION OF ABNORMAL SEXUAL DEVELOPMENT

The disorders of abnormal sexual differentiation can be delineated in several ways. We prefer to place affected individuals initially into one of several broad categories that can be identified readily on the basis of chromosomal complement or gonadal status: gonadal dysgenesis, Klinefelter syndrome, true hermaphroditism, sex-reversed (XX) males, female pseudohermaphroditism, and male pseudohermaphroditism. Related categories include anomalies limited to müllerian or wolffian derivatives and forms of hypogonadism occurring in individuals with normal external genitalia. Within each category are various disorders that must be distinguished from one another. An etiologic classification is the traditional way

Birth Defects: Original Article Series, Volume XII, Number 1, pages 15–50

of delineating dysmorphic states,[1] and the disorders of abnormal sexual differentiation can be approached in a similar fashion. Some investigators prefer a classification based solely upon a patient's endocrine status. For example, male pseudohermaphroditism might be delineated into testicular biosynthetic, testicular metabolic, androgen insensitive, or otherwise unexplained androgen sensitive disorders. While theoretically appealing, a purely endocrine delineation is, in 1975, impractical because 1) there are too many overlapping areas between various disorders, and 2) relatively few disorders have been investigated thoroughly enough to warrant the appropriate categorization. In a forthcoming monograph[2] almost all reported disorders of abnormal sexual differentiation will be considered. In this communication only selected disorders will be discussed.

OVARIAN NEOPLASIA

The apparent annual incidence of ovarian cancer varies from less than 5/100,000 persons/year in Chile, Japan and South Africa to slightly greater than 10/100,000 in Colombia, Canada, Israel, and the United States.[3] Of all gynecologic malignancies 15–25% are ovarian[4,5]; 25% of ovarian tumors are malignant.[4] Ovarian carcinoma occurs most frequently during the 7th and 8th decades; in those years the prevalence is 10 times greater than during the first 3 decades (Fig. 1). The probability that an ovarian tumor is malignant is highest if it is detected in an older person.[6] Deaths from ovarian cancer in the United States range from less than 1/100,000 females under 20 years to nearly 40/100,000 females over age 70.[7]

Ovarian tumors are classified by histogenesis: germinal epithelium, germ cell, or sex cord-mesenchyme (Table 1). Ninety percent of ovarian tumors arise from the germinal epithelium, the mesothelial surface of the ovary (Table 2). Most

TABLE 1. Simplified Classification of Ovarian Tumors Based Upon Histogenesis

A. Tumors of germinal epithelial origin (mesothelium)

Serous	Mesonephroid (clear cell)
Mucinous	Brenner
Endometrioid	Mixed forms

B. Tumors of germ-cell origin

Dysgerminoma	Choriocarcinoma
Embryonal carcinoma	Gonadoblastoma (also contains sex
Teratoma	cord-mesenchyme derivatives)
Mixed forms	

C. Tumors of sex cord-mesenchyme origin (gonadal stroma)

Granulosa cell	Sertoli cell
Theca cell	Leydig cell
Mixed forms	

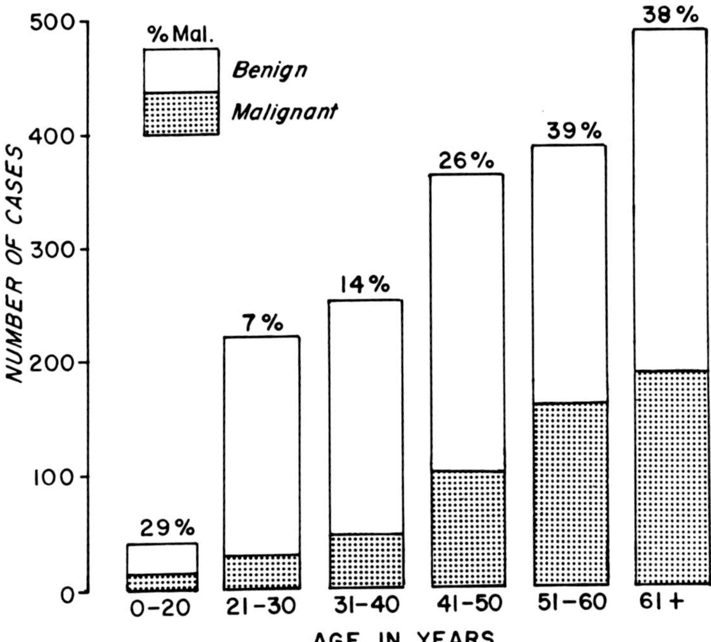

Fig. 1. Comparison of the frequencies of benign and malignant ovarian tumors at different ages. The figure above each bar indicates the percentage of malignant tumors in that particular age group. Modified from data presented by Fathalla,[6] based upon 1734 consecutively ascertained tumors.

germinal epithelial tumors are serous, mucinous, endometrioid, or mesonephroid.[8] Germ-cell tumors are classified into 4 groups: dysgerminoma, embryonal carcinoma, choriocarcinoma, and teratoma.[9-11] Epithelial tumors, either benign or malignant, are the most common ovarian tumors in normal adult women, but they are relatively rare in patients under 15 years (Table 3) and in patients with abnormal sexual differentiation.[12-15] Therefore, in our summary of ovarian tumors we will emphasize germ-cell tumors and stromal cell (sex cord-mesenchyme) tumors, and only briefly discuss epithelial tumors.

GERM-CELL TUMORS

Dysgerminoma

Dysgerminomas are characterized by large oval gonocytes that contain dark nuclei and clear cytoplasm; these cells are arranged in a delicate connective tissue matrix infiltrated by lymphocytes (Fig. 2). Dysgerminomas often contain

TABLE 2. Relative Frequencies of Some Ovarian Tumors*

Benign serous	16%
Malignant serous	6
Benign mucinous	18
Malignant mucinous	6
Benign teratoma	20
Malignant teratoma	1
Fibrothecoma	6
Granulosa-theca	3
Dysgerminoma	2
Embryonal carcinoma	1
Brenner tumor	1

*Metastatic carcinomas, unspecified types of tumors, and tumors with a frequency of less than 1% are not listed.
(Adapted from Norris, H. J. and Chorlton, I: Functioning tumors of the ovary. Clin. Obstet. Gynecol. 17:189, 1974.)

TABLE 3. Relative Frequencies of Ovarian Tumors in Individuals Under Age 15 Years[13]

A. Germ-cell tumors		71%
Benign teratoma	13%	
Malignant teratoma	25	
Dysgerminoma	17	
Embryonal carcinoma	16	
B. Germinal epithelial tumors		6%
C. Sex cord-mesenchyme tumors		19%
Granulosa cell	5%	
Fibrothecoma	4	
Sertoli-Leydig cell	3	
Nonspecific	7	
D. Others		4%

(Adapted from Norris, H. J. and Jensen, R. D.: Relative frequency of ovarian neoplasms in children and adolescents. Cancer 30:713, 1972.)

other neoplastic germ-cell components.[4] Ovarian dysgerminomas and testicular seminomas are histologically identical; however, dysgerminomas usually arise early in the 3rd decade, whereas seminomas usually arise later.[16] Dysgerminomas are quite sensitive to irradiation, and in selected cases an 82.8% five-year survival has been reported.[17] Gross appearance, presence of metastases, and presence of other germ-cell components influence prognosis.[4,18]

Embryonal Carcinoma

Embryonal carcinomas are characterized by embryoid or Schiller-Duval bodies, which resemble a glomerulus (mesonephroma ovarii) — a central vascular tuft is surrounded by a cystic space lined by small flat cells (Fig. 3). Some investigators consider embryonal carcinoma too general a term.[19] Because the histologic pattern is reminiscent of the endodermal sinus in rodent placentas, the term endodermal sinus tumor is favored by many pathologists. However, as there is no endodermal sinus in the human placenta still others prefer the term yolk sac tumor. Embryonal carcinomas may arise in infants or in adults (mean age of onset 18 years). About 100 cases have been reported.

Gaillard[20] believes that embryonal carcinomas also contain extraembryonic tissue of entoblastic or mesoblastic origin. Several subtypes may exist.[21] Embryonal carcinomas are highly malignant, and, in contrast to dysgerminomas, are unresponsive to irradiation.[22]

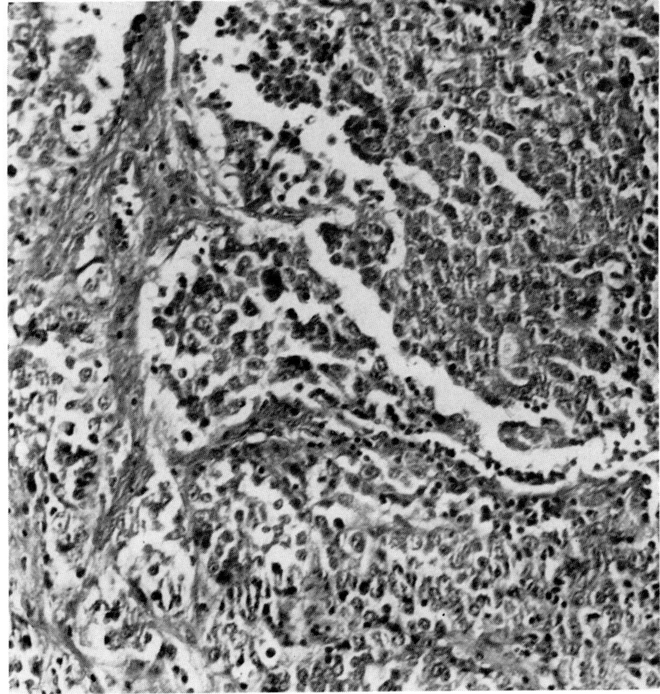

Fig. 2. An ovarian dysgerminoma. Germ cells lie within a delicate connective tissue stroma infiltrated by lymphocytes. A seminoma is similar in appearance (X 175).

Teratoma

Teratomas contain cells derived from more than one of the 3 germ layers: ectoderm, endoderm, mesoderm. They may arise in gonadal or in extragonadal sites, but we shall consider only gonadal teratomas.

Ovarian teratomas (dermoid tumors) probably arise by parthenogenesis.[23] The various germ layer components vary in degree of maturation, sometimes being immature and sometimes being mature, eg containing skin appendages or cartilage (Fig. 4). The most common component is squamous epithelium, and this is also the component most likely to be malignant. Ninety-eight percent of ovarian teratomas are benign,[24] in contrast to testicular teratomas, which are often malignant. Nearly one half of ovarian tumors occurring in the first 2 decades are teratomas.[10,25] Within a cystic ovarian teratoma lies a prominence called the dermoid process (Rokitansky protuberance or mammilla), in which malignant cells are most likely to be found. One to 2% of apparently benign cystic teratomas contain a malignant focus.[4] Solid teratomas are malignant more frequently

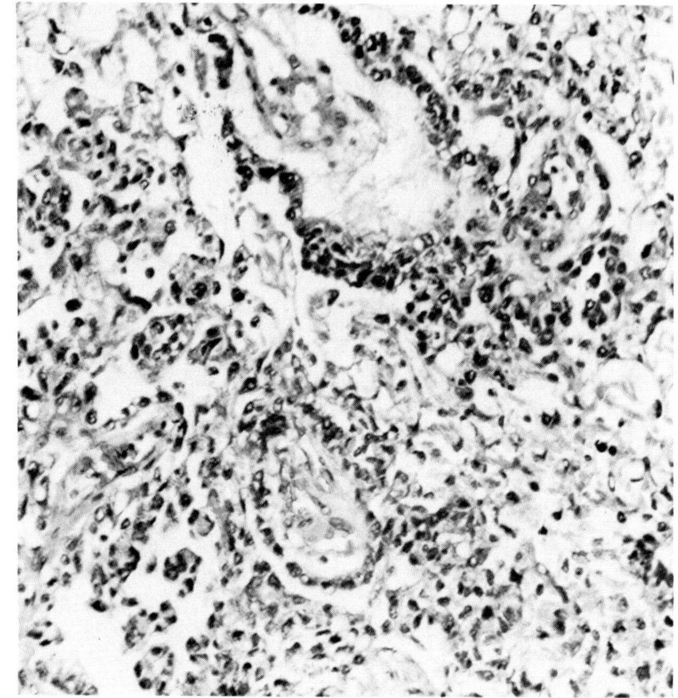

Fig. 3. An ovarian embryonal carcinoma. Schiller-Duval bodies are present within loose stroma. These bodies resemble a glomerulus — a central vessel is surrounded by a sinusoidal space lined by small flat cells. A testicular embryonal carcinoma is similar in appearance (X 175).

than cystic tumors, but malignancy cannot be predicted on the basis of gross appearance alone.

Gonadoblastoma

Gonadoblastomas arise almost exclusively in dysgenetic gonads of 46,XY individuals. According to Scully,[26] a gonadoblastoma contains 2 kinds of cells: 1) primitive germ cells, and 2) sex-cord (Sertoli-granulosa) cells (Fig. 5). For diagnosis Teter prefers the additional presence of Leydig or theca-lutein cells[27]; if present, he refers to such a tumor as gonocytoma III. However, Scully believes that Leydig cells occur only in postpuberal patients, hence their presence is age-dependent. Hyaline bodies and calcified areas are usually present, and can be detected by roentgenograms.

Gonadoblastomas may contain an area of dysgerminoma. Scully reported stromal invasion by the dysgerminoma component in one half of such mixed tumors.

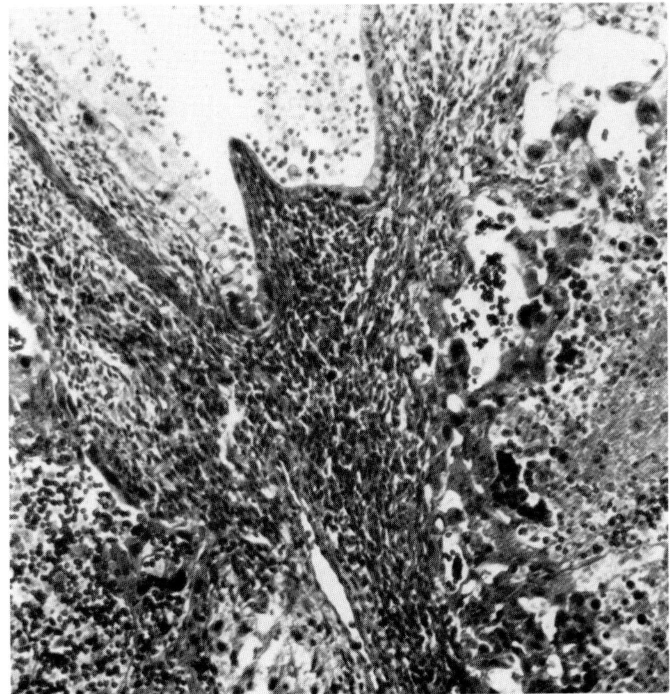

Fig. 4. A malignant ovarian teratoma. Benign glandular epithelium is present in the upper left portion; adjacent to this are anaplastic changes (X 175).

In 6 of 74 cases (8.1%),[26] a gonadoblastoma was associated with yet other germ-cell tumors: embryonal teratoma, embryonal carcinoma, endodermal sinus tumor, or choriocarcinoma. Talerman likewise estimated that about 10% of gonadoblastomas are associated with a more malignant germ-cell tumor, an occurrence that adversely affects prognosis.[28] Finally, a gonadoblastoma can synthesize estrogens or androgens, hence feminization or virilization may occur.

SEX CORD-MESENCHYME TUMORS

Granulosa cell tumors, theca cell tumors, Sertoli cell tumors, and Leydig cell tumors, all of which occur individually or in combination, are derived from the sex cords or the mesenchyme of the embryonic gonad. Thus, Scully prefers the term sex cord-mesenchyme tumors.[29] These tumors can synthesize hormones that feminize or virilize. Sex cord-mesenchyme tumors, particularly granulosa cell tumors, are the most common ovarian tumors in domestic animals,[30] but they are relatively rare in humans.

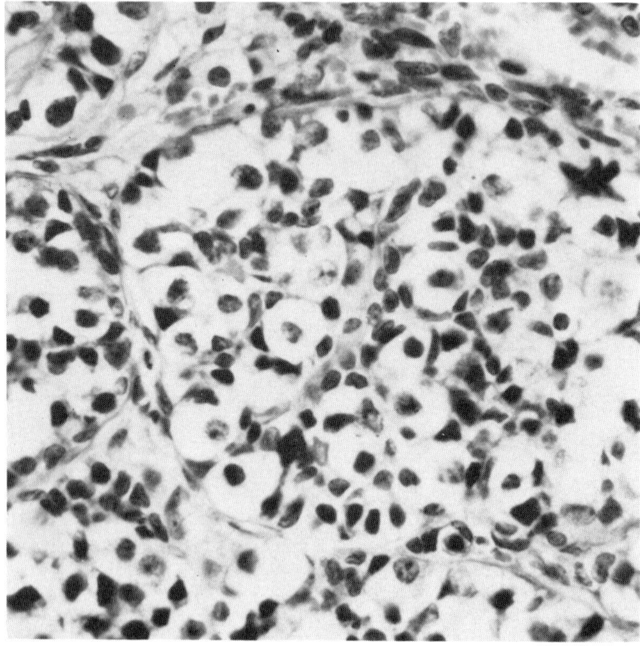

Fig. 5. A gonadoblastoma, present in male with persistent müllerian derivatives. Primitive germ cells and Sertoli-granulosa-like cells are present (× 490). From German and Morillo-Cucci.[137]

Granulosa Cell Tumors

Granulosa cell tumors consist of granulosa cells that may be arranged in folliculoid, cylindroid, pseudoadenomatoid, or sarcomatoid patterns. The follicular pattern is most common, but multiple varieties may occur in a single tumor. In a follicular pattern a central core of eosinophilic-staining material is surrounded by granulosa cells; this complex is called a Call-Exner body (Fig. 6). In pure granulosa cell tumors the mean age is 50 years,[31,32] yet in one series of 92 patients there were 5 premenarchal patients, 2 of whom developed precocious puberty.[31] Fox believes that all granulosa cell tumors should be considered potentially malignant because within 20 years 50% of affected individuals will die of their tumor.[31]

Sertoli-Leydig Cell Tumors

Sertoli cells are derived from male sex cord cells. In combination with Leydig cells, Sertoli cells may form a testicular-like adenoma within the ovary, as originally described by Pick.[33] Too few ovarian Sertoli-Leydig cell tumors have been

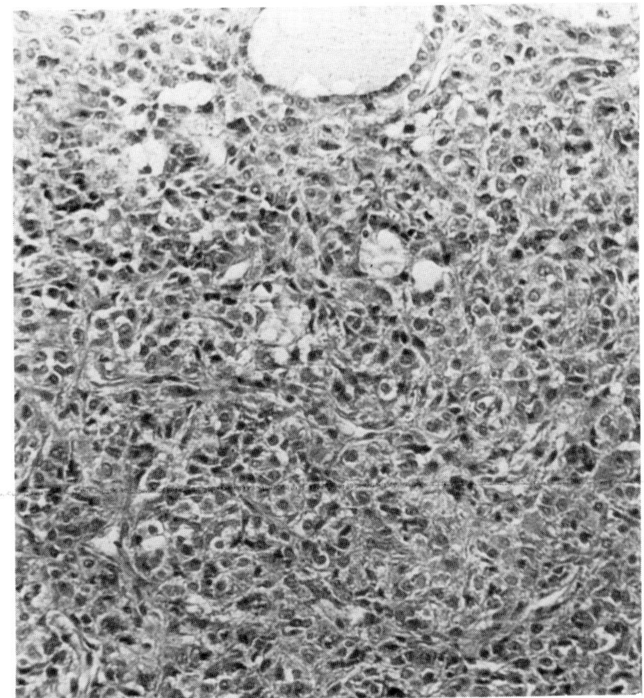

Fig. 6. An ovarian granulosa cell tumor. Granulosa cells are polyhedral in shape and form rosette-like patterns around cystic spaces. These complexes, termed Call-Exner bodies, resemble primordial follicles but do not contain germ cells (X 175).

reported to predict accurately the malignant potential; malignancy rates of 5–30% have been estimated.[28]

Thecomas and Leydig Cell Tumors

Several mesenchyme tumors — theca cell tumors and Leydig cell tumors — constitute the remainder of ovarian sex cord-mesenchyme tumors. The mesenchyme is a pluripotential cellular matrix that during embryogenesis separates entoderm from ectoderm; some mesenchymal cells differentiate into ovarian stromal cells, which in turn give rise to theca cells and Leydig cells. Thus, theca cell tumors and Leydig cell tumors are sometimes called stromal cell tumors. Sternberg and Roth believe that theca cell tumors and Leydig cell tumors arise from mature ovarian stroma, and, further, that Leydig cell tumors can arise from hilar cells.[34] Thecomas are frequently associated with granulosa cells; such a tumor is designated granulosa-theca cell tumor. Theca cell tumors, which are usually benign,[35] can be distinguished from fibromas only by fat stains. Leydig cell tumors are also usually benign.

EPITHELIAL TUMORS

Brenner tumors and mucinous tumors are the final ovarian tumors we shall discuss. Three mucinous cystadenomas and 2 Brenner tumors were the only epithelial tumors noted in one tabulation of tumors occurring in patients with abnormal sexual development.[12] All 3 mucinous tumors were in true hermaphrodites; one Brenner tumor also occurred in a true hermaphrodite, whereas the other was in a patient with gonadal dysgenesis.

Brenner tumors are characterized by aggregates of polyhedral cells with large, ovoid, grooved (coffee bean-shaped) nuclei. These aggregates, which may undergo cystic degeneration, are surrounded by a fibrous stroma. Mucinous cells are frequently detected in Brenner tumors. Brenner tumors may arise directly from the germinal epithelium or from Walthard cells, which themselves might have arisen from the germinal epithelium.[36] Teilum[17] has reviewed the histogenesis. Ninety-eight to 99% of Brenner tumors are benign,[37] and there is no consistent clinical pattern.[38]

Mucinous cystadenomas, relatively common tumors, are frequently large and multicystic. The cyst walls are lined with tall columnar cells containing clear cytoplasm and basal nuclei. Mucinous and serous cystadenomas comprise most ovarian epithelial tumors.

TESTICULAR NEOPLASIA

Testicular tumors occur in about 2–2.5/100,000 males/year in the United States and Canada,[39,40] and they account for 0.64% of all male oncologic deaths. They occur less often among American and African blacks than among whites.[41–43] Ninety-four percent of testicular tumors originate from germ cells; the remainder originate from the gonadal stroma, which arises from mesenchyme.

GERM-CELL TESTICULAR TUMORS

There are 4 kinds of germ-cell tumors: seminomas, embryonal carcinomas, choriocarcinomas, and teratomas; however, 40% of germ-cell tumors contain 2 or more cell types. Testicular tumors occur most frequently in infants, young adults (20–35 years), and older adults (50 years and over).[40] Seminomas are rare in infancy, whereas teratomas and embryonal cell carcinomas are relatively common. In young adults all varieties can occur with similar frequencies. In older adults seminomas are most frequent.

Seminomas

Seminomas are characterized by large cells with clear cytoplasm that exists in a delicate fibrovascular stroma infiltrated with lymphocytes; this pattern is reminiscent of ovarian dysgerminomas (Fig. 2). Seminomas, which account for one third to two thirds of testicular tumors, are divided into spermatocytic and anaplastic varieties. Spermatocytic seminomas, which occur in older men, are associated with a 90–95% five-year survival; anaplastic seminomas have a worse prognosis.

Embryonal Carcinoma

Testicular embryonal carcinomas contain large pleomorphic anaplastic embryonic cells that exist in one of several patterns: acinar, tubular, papillary, endodermal sinus, and solid. The endodermal sinus variety is the most frequent testicular tumor in children.[44] It resembles an ovarian embryonal carcinoma because Schiller-Duval bodies are present, ie a cystic space containing a vascular tuft is surrounded by epithelial cells and myxomatous stroma (see Fig. 3). An estimated 5-year survival is 20–30% for tumors occurring in adults and 70% for tumors occurring in infants.[40]

Choriocarcinoma

Choriocarcinomas contain cytotrophoblastic cells and syncytiotrophoblastic cells. These tumors occur primarily in the 2nd and 3rd decades. A pure form is rare. Choriocarcinomas synthesize human chorionic gonadotropin (HCG), assay of which can be used to diagnose the disorder and to monitor treatment.[45] Prognosis for this rare tumor is relatively poor.

Teratoma

Teratomas contain at least 2 of the 3 germ layers: ectoderm, mesoderm, endoderm. These components may be benign or malignant. Teratomas comprise only 9% of adult testicular tumors, but they are the second most common childhood testicular tumor.[46]

STROMAL CELL TUMORS

The most common stromal cell tumors are Leydig cell tumors and Sertoli cell tumors, representative cells of which may coexist in a single tumor. Theca-granulosa cell tumors and primitive gonadal stromal tumors have also been reported. Stromal cell tumors usually occur in children.

Leydig Cell Tumors

Leydig cells are polygonal-shaped cells that synthesize testosterone and occasionally contain cytoplasmic crystals (Reinke crystalloids). Leydig cell tumors, rarely malignant, often masculinize affected individuals, but they may also feminize or have no hormonal effect.[47]

Sertoli Cell Tumors

Sertoli cell tumors contain cells with abundant cytoplasm that are arranged in tubular-like fashion. They are usually not malignant.[48]

CRYPTORCHIDISM AND ITS RELATION TO TESTICULAR TUMORS

A testis that fails to descend into the scrotum by birth is cryptorchid. Normally, both testes have migrated into the scrotum by the 8th month of intrauterine development. At birth 97.3% of full-term infants and 79% of premature infants have scrotal testes.[49] Nine months after birth 99.2% of infants have scrotal testes.[49] Testes that fail to descend after 9 months often never descend, as evidenced by observations that 99.2–99.8% of males undergoing examination for induction into the military have scrotal testes.[50] Three fourths of cryptorchid testes are inguinal; one fourth are abdominal.

Etiology of Cryptorchidism

The etiology of cryptorchidism is unknown. Genetic factors, endocrine factors, and anatomic abnormalities are important. That 4% of cryptorchid males have an affected relative suggests the importance of genetic factors.[51] The incidence of cryptorchidism varies also according to the species, further suggesting genetic control of testicular descent. Birds, reptiles, elephants, whales, and several other animals normally have undescended testes.[52]

Histologic Aspects

Three phases of postnatal testicular development can be defined: 1) resting phase – birth to 4 years; 2) growth phase – 4 to 10 years; and 3) developmental phase – 10 years through adolescence.[53–55] A cryptorchid testis resembles the normal testis until 4 to 5 years; thereafter, Sertoli cell development ceases, seminiferous tubules fail to mature, and peritubular fibrosis occurs.

Are cryptorchid testes histologically abnormal because the testes differentiate abnormally (dysgenetic testes), or are the histologic changes merely secondary to an unfavorable (eg intraabdominal) environment?[56–58] Both factors are probably important. First, spermatogenesis is commonly known to be arrested in cryptorchid testes. On the other hand, Sohval reported that about one half of cryptorchid patients, 10 years or older and without apparent endocrine or genital abnormalities, have a dysgenetic testis.[56] The following changes could reflect abnormal differentiation: 1) after puberty immature seminiferous tubules contain undifferentiated stromal cells rather than mature Sertoli cells; 2) sometimes no Sertoli cells, no Leydig cells, or no spermatogonia are present; and 3) histologically abnormal cryptorchid testes are resistant to sclerosis, whereas histologically normal cryptorchid testes are not.[56] Salle confirmed many of these findings.[57] In addition, testicular dysgenesis has been described in the contralateral, normally descended testis of unilaterally cryptorchid men.[56] Also, about 25% of men who undergo prepuberal orchiopexy subsequently are infertile.[59,60] One way to test the hypothesis that cryptorchid testes usually have differentiated abnormally would be to study the chromosomal complement of testicular tissue derived from cryptorchid but otherwise normal males. Chromosomal abnormalities would suggest testicular dysgenesis. Furthermore, if chromosomal abnormalities were limited to the testes, lymphocytes would be chromosomally normal. One such study,[51] which purported to show a high incidence of chromosomal abnormalities (usually an additional or a missing group C chromosome), has indeed been reported; however, additional documentation is needed.

RISK OF NEOPLASIA IN CRYPTORCHID TESTES

The probability that a cryptorchid testis will undergo malignant transformation is unknown, but it is at least 14 times greater than for normally descended testes.[40] About 11% of males with testicular neoplasia have been or are cryptorchid.[40,61] Interestingly, orchiopexy does not eliminate the risk of neoplasia, particularly if performed after 6 years of age. For example, Gehring et al reported that one third of cryptorchid-associated carcinoma occurred following orchiopexy.[62] Dow et al reported 73 cryptorchid-associated malignancies in 2100 testicular tumors; 14 of the 73 patients had undergone orchiopexy, but none prior to 6 years of age.[63] These observations notwithstanding, only a few cases of neoplasia have occurred in individuals in whom orchiopexy was performed prior to 10 years of age.

The increased risk of neoplasia in cryptorchid testes could be explained in either of 2 ways: 1) the same factor(s) that cause cryptorchidism also cause neoplasia, or 2) an intraabdominal or inguinal environment is oncogenic per se, irrespective of the factors that lead to cryptorchidism. Probably the former is more important. This would be consistent with observations that many cryptorchid testes are dysgenetic.[56] Sohval detected dysgenetic changes in the testes of 5 out of 42 patients with testicular tumors; 4 of the 5 were cryptorchid.[64] Significantly, in 20% of patients with unilateral cryptorchidism and testicular neoplasia, the malignancy arises in the contralateral scrotal testis.[65]

A second possibility is that prolonged exposure to an intraabdominal environment is oncogenic for testes, irrespective of the factors that cause cryptorchidism. Perhaps the increased intraabdominal temperature adversely affects metabolic function and nucleic acid synthesis. Indeed, in guinea pigs, testicular development is delayed if descent is experimentally arrested; however, subsequent orchiopexy permits active spermatogenesis.[66] Further support for this theory can be derived from observations that testicular neoplasia occurs in about 5% of males with testicular feminization or with persistence of müllerian derivatives (see below); in neither disorder is testicular differentiation abnormal. This theory cannot, however, readily explain a) the increased incidence of neoplasia in men who previously underwent orchiopexy, or b) the increased incidence of neoplasia in the contralateral scrotal testis of cryptorchid men. The former might be explained by hypothesizing that both testicular dysgenesis and an abnormal environment act synergistically to induce neoplastic transformation. In particular, the risk of neoplasia remains increased if the testis remains in an intraabdominal environment during the growth phase, 4–10 years of age. The occurrence of neoplasia in the contralateral scrotal testis (the latter theory) might be explained by postulating that an apparently normally descended testis was actually once an unrecognized cryptorchid testis that underwent spontaneous descent at puberty.

Although the relationship between cryptorchidism and testicular carcinoma remains unclear, some clinical recommendations can, nonetheless, be offered. Orchiopexy performed after the testicular growth phase (4–10 years) does not eliminate the risk of neoplasia; it may not even decrease the risk. Moreover, a dysgenetic testis has a greatly reduced fertility potential. Therefore, we recommend that orchiectomy be considered in any patient who presents after 6–10 years of age with a dysgenetic unilateral cryptorchid testis.

SURVEY OF DISORDERS OF SEXUAL DIFFERENTIATION

Gonadal Dysgenesis

Individuals with gonadal dysgenesis have streaks of connective tissue lacking germ cells — streak gonads (Fig. 7). Pituitary gonadotropin levels are increased; estrogen levels are decreased. Patients with gonadal dysgenesis may be short in stature and have certain somatic anomalies, in which case the Turner stigmata are said to be present.[67] Gonadal dysgenesis is usually associated with monosomy for the X chromosome or structural rearrangements of the X or Y chromosome — a cytogenetic etiology. However, gonadal dysgenesis may also be associated with apparently normal male (46, XY) or female (46,XX) complements — a genetic etiology.[68]

The term most frequently applied to individuals with gonadal dysgenesis is "Turner's syndrome." Unfortunately, "Turner's syndrome" does not connote identical features to all investigators. For this reason we prefer to apply the term "gonadal dysgenesis" to all individuals with streak gonads, reserving the term "Turner stigmata" for individuals with short stature and certain other somatic anomalies.

Cytogenetic Forms 45,X and Variants Without a Y

If gonadal dysgenesis is associated with a complement lacking a Y chromosome (eg 45,X; 45,X/46,XX; 46,X, del(XP); 45,X,i(Xq)), tumors are rarely present. For example, Simpson recently reviewed 232 cases of 45,X, 69 cases of 45,X/46,XX, 26 cases of Xp deletions, 20 cases of Xq deletions, 5 cases of 46,X,i(Xp), and 22 cases of 45,X,i(Xq).[67] None of the individuals surveyed had

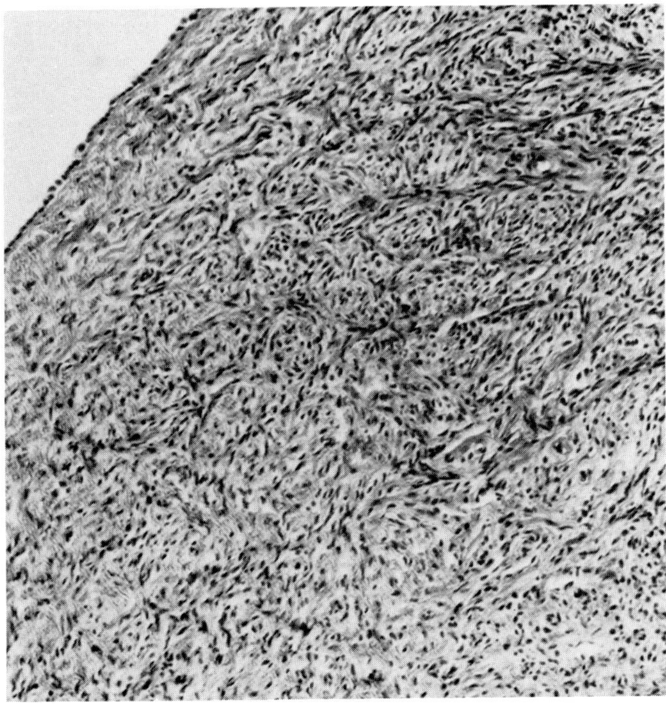

Fig. 7. A streak gonad. The germinal epithelium can be identified in the upper left. No germ cells are present (X 175).

a gonadal tumor. These data indicate that elevated gonadotropin levels per se are not associated with an increased risk of gonadal neoplasia.

On the other hand, Wertelecki et al studied 289 patients with the Turner stigmata for the presence of nongonadal tumors; cytogenetic studies were not always performed.[69] One patient had a hilar cell adenoma, and 8 patients had a nongonadal tumor — 3 of neural origin, 3 of gastrointestinal origin, one carcinoma of the thyroid, and one leukemia. Other investigators have not commented upon a possible increased risk for nongonadal neoplasia. However, various hamartomatous growths — pigmented nevi, gastrointestinal telangiectasias, capillary hemangiomas — are associated with 45,X, hence a relationship between 45,X and nongonadal neoplasia is conceivable.

Endometrial carcinoma has been reported in 45,X patients treated with diethylstilbestrol.[70, 71] These patients usually had been treated for many years prior to onset of neoplasia. Interestingly, the tumor was often adenosquamous carcinoma, rather than the more common adenocarcinoma. These cases nothwithstanding , the prevalence of carcinoma in estrogen-treated 45,X patients is relatively low; thus, hormone replacement should not be withheld.

45,X/46,XY and Related Complements

45,X/46,XY patients may have bilateral streak gonads, but more often they have ambiguous external genitalia and either bilateral dysgenetic testes or a unilateral testis and a contralateral streak gonad.[72] Thus, 45,X/46,XY mosaicism is most appropriately considered as a form of male pseudohermaphroditism (see below). Ten to 15% of 45,X/46,XY patients develop gonadal tumors.

Genetic Forms

Gonadal dysgenesis is usually associated with an abnormal chromosomal complement. However, occasionally patients with streak gonads histologically similar to that found in chromosomally abnormal individuals have an apparently normal female (46, XX) or male (46, XY) complement.

XX Gonadal Dysgenesis. This condition results from a mutant autosomal recessive gene.[68] Most affected patients are of normal stature and lack somatic anomalies. However, the prevalence of neurosensory deafness is increased in some familial aggregates; thus, two forms may exist — one with and one without deafness. No patient has developed a gonadal tumor, although one developed adenocarcinoma of the endometrium.[68]

XY Gonadal Dysgenesis (Swyer Syndrome). This condition results from an X-linked recessive or a male-limited autosomal dominant gene. Affected patients are normal in stature and lack the somatic anomalies comprising the Turner stigmata. The streak gonads in XY gonadal dysgenesis are identical histologically to those present in 45,X gonadal dysgenesis; however, in XY gonadal dysgenesis gonadoblastomas and dysgerminomas are frequently associated. The probability that a gonadal tumor, usually a gonadoblastoma or a dysgerminoma, will arise in a patient with XY gonadal dysgenesis appears to be about 20–30%[26, 68, 73] although available data are retrospective and thus potentially biased. These germ-cell tumors arise at a relatively early age, often in the first decade, unlike neoplasia occurring in cryptorchid testes. Pure gonadoblastomas are probably benign, but they may be associated with malignant germ-cell tumors like dysgerminomas. Thus, patients with XY gonadal dysgenesis should be offered gonadal extirpation soon after their diagnosis.

The prevalence of tumors is higher in familial cases than in nonfamilial cases. Among the 26 reported familial cases of XY gonadal dysgenesis are 15 individuals who either had a gonadoblastoma, a dysgerminoma, or both[74–85]; several individuals had bilateral tumors. In a 1971 review of 45 nonfamilial cases, Simpson et al tabulated 11 cases of gonadal tumors (24%).[68] The age of onset and the clinical behavior of the tumors seem to be about the same if the tumor originated in a nonfamilial case as in a familial case. Tumors have also been present in about

30% of XY gonadal dysgenesis patients who were ascertained because of amenorrhea and who had been routinely explored surgically.[27, 85–89] Thus, by either of these 2 approaches — retrospective surveys or prospectively explored patients — the risk of neoplasia seems to be at least 20–30%. This risk is higher than that for normal males with a cryptorchid testis.

Why is XY gonadal dysgenesis associated with an increased probability of neoplastic transformation? We might consider 2 general explanations: 1) Poorly differentiated gonadal tissue, specifically the type present in patients with XY gonadal dysgenesis, has a propensity for neoplastic transformation, irrespective of the factors that produced the dysgenetic gonads — genetic, cytogenetic, or teratogenic. 2) The gene that produces XY gonadal dysgenesis not only causes germ-cell absence but also confers a propensity for neoplastic transformation, ie gonadal hypoplasia and neoplasia are etiologically related phenomena.

1) The increased prevalence of neoplasia might reflect the existence of poorly differentiated XY gonadal tissue in an intraabdominal position, subject to heat, elevated gonadotropin levels, and possibly other endogenous factors. This hypothesis is supported by observations that the prevalence of gonadal neoplasia is also increased in 45,X/46,XY mosaicism,[72] the etiology of which is not genetic but cytogenetic. It is relevant that during embryonic development XY germ cells divide more rapidly than XX germ cells.[90] Thus, dysgenetic XY germ cells, originally scheduled to exist in the scrotum at a cooler temperature, and thus presumably at a lower metabolic rate, might respond to an intraabdominal position with an increased metabolic rate; thus, the propensity for neoplastic transformation might be increased.

2) The mutant gene for XY gonadal dysgenesis might more directly confer an increased propensity for neoplastic transformation. This hypothesis is supported by the early age of neoplasia and the relatively high frequency of bilateral tumors, both well-known characteristics of heritable tumors.[91] Fibroblasts of XY gonadal dysgenesis patients, but not 45,X patients, also show increased susceptibility to transformation following exposure to Simian Papovavirus-40 (SV40).[92] This suggests that the XY gonadal dysgenesis mutant not only causes streak gonads but also increases the susceptibility of those gonads to undergo neoplastic transformation. The manner in which the mutant gene exerts its propensity for neoplasia is unknown. However, at least 3 related possibilities might be offered:

a) The mutant gene causes aneuploidy. The aneuploidy, which in XY gonadal dysgenesis might usually be limited to sex chromosomes of germ cells, might sometimes involve other chromosomes and lead to a neoplastic clone. This idea would be especially attractive if the gene produced aneuploidy by initially causing chromosomal breakage.

b) A hypothesis not necessarily mutually exclusive from the following paragraph (c) is that the mutant gene alters cell-surface antigens in embryonic germ cells.[93–96] Bennett and colleagues have made some observations that are relevant to this question.[93-96] In mice there are a series of at least 5 recessive genes at the T locus. Homozygosity for each allele produces a specific group of anomalies that results in embryonic death. Mice homozygous for one of these alleles, t^{W18}, show massive overgrowth of primitive streak cells prior to embryonic death.[93] Artzt and Bennett transplanted portions of the overgrown primitive streak of homozygous embryos (t^{W18}/t^{W18}) to testes of fathers, single uncles, and double uncles.[93] Fifteen of 46 t^{W18}/t^{W18} transplants produced malignant growths, whereas embryonic transplants from normal littermates produced only a few benign teratomas. Subsequent studies revealed that embryonic tissue and sperm of t^{W18} homozygotes lacked a cell-surface antigen present in normal mice. Thus, cells that differentiated abnormally as result of lacking a cell-surface antigen were associated with neoplastic transformation. A similar phenomenon could be postulated for XY gonadal dysgenesis.

c) More generally, perhaps the mutant gene represents the first step in a two-step sequence responsible for tumorigenesis, utilizing the scheme of Knudson et al.[91] The second step might be a somatic mutation, an environmental agent, or a cytogenetic error of the type alluded to above. A two-step hypothesis is consistent with observations that the tumor prevalence is higher in XY gonadal dysgenesis (20–30%) than in 45,X/46,XY (10–15%); the former might require only one step, the latter two.

KLINEFELTER SYNDROME

Males with at least one Y chromosome and at least 2 X chromosomes have the Klinefelter syndrome. The most characteristic feature is seminiferous tubule dysgenesis, ie atrophy and hyalinization of the seminiferous tubules, and a relative increase in the number of Leydig cells. Gonadotropin levels are increased and androgen levels are decreased. About 20% of 47,XXY patients have visibly evident gynecomastia, although a higher percentage have palpable parenchymal breast tissue.[97] Somatic anomalies and mental retardation occur in only a small proportion of 47,XXY individuals, but they are invariably present in 48,XXXY or 49,XXXXY individuals.[98,99]

Gonadal tumors rarely arise in patients with the Klinefelter syndrome, regardless of their chromosomal complement. Analogous to 45,X gonadal dysgenesis, this probably indicates that increased gonadotropin levels per se are not oncogenic. However, Gustavson et al reported bilateral teratomas in each of 2 nontwin 47,XXY sibs.[100]

On the other hand, the prevalence of breast carcinoma is higher in 47,XXY males than in 46,XY males.[101-103] Three to 4% of males with carcinoma of the breast have the Klinefelter syndrome; this incidence is about one fifth that of normal females and about 20 times greater than that of normal males.[103] Decreased androgens per se are probably not of primary importance in the etiology of breast carcinoma in males because the prevalence of breast carcinoma is not increased in males with hypogonadotropic hypogonadism. The association of elevated gonadotropin with decreased androgens might be important. Prolactin levels are not increased in the Klinefelter syndrome.[104]

Leukemia has been associated with the Klinefelter syndrome,[105] but whether its association is more than coincidental is unknown. Likewise, Coley et al reported an interesting case of a 47,XXY man who developed 6 primary neoplasias, 5 malignant.[106] That these observations may be more than coincidental is suggested by 1) observations that 47,XXY fibroblasts display increased susceptibility to transformation following exposure to SV40 virus,[107] and 2) suggestions that Klinefelter patients have an increased frequency of asthma,[108] a disease that might have an immunologic basis; thus, Klinefelter patients might be incapable of a normal immunologic response.

TRUE HERMAPHRODITISM

True hermaphrodites have ovarian as well as testicular tissue. To warrant the diagnosis an affected individual should have 1) histologically verified ovarian follicles or proof of their prior existence (eg corpora albicantia), not simply fibrous stroma, and 2) seminiferous tubules or spermatozoa, not simply Leydig cells. Testicular tubules are usually atrophic and hyalinized; by contrast, ovarian follicles are frequently well developed. At puberty most true hermaphrodites develop breasts and remain poorly virilized.[109]

About two thirds of true hermaphrodites are 46,XX; the remainder are usually 46,XX/46,XY, 46,XX/47,XXY, or 46,XY.[109] 46,XX/46,XY and 46,XX/47,XXY true hermaphrodites, and, we suspect, perhaps most 46,XY true hermaphrodites result from chimerism or mosaicism. Some 46,XX true hermaphrodites could result from chimerism, X-Y interchange, or Y-autosome translocation, but many may result from a sex-reversal gene, such as Sxr in mice.[110] Because true hermaphrodites have different complements, it would be preferable to consider neoplasia in terms of the complement of affected individuals. Unfortunately, most cases associated with neoplasia have not been cytogenetically investigated.

The incidence of gonadal neoplasia in true hermaphrodites appears to be low.[109] Neoplasia has been reported only once in over 100 cases of 46,XX true hermaphrodites,[109] only once in 23 cases of 46,XY true hermaphrodites,[111] and in none of 18 cases of 46,XX/46,XY true hermaphrodites (see Simpson[2] for derivation of samples). In the precytogenetic era 7 true hermaphrodites had gonadal neoplasia.[112–118] Four tumors were ovarian and 3 were testicular. The only malignant tumors were testicular in origin. That testicular but not ovarian malignancy has occurred might reflect the fact that testicular tissue is usually not as well-differentiated as ovarian tissue (see above). One would also expect testes of true hermaphrodites to be affected adversely by their usual intra-abdominal position. In fact, perhaps the occurrence of testicular tumors in true hermaphrodites merely reflects the intraabdominal environment. At any rate, a factor other than abnormal germ-cell differentiation per se must be postulated, because otherwise both ovarian and testicular malignancy would occur with equal frequency.

Two true hermaphrodites have developed carcinoma of the breast.[109,119]

SEX-REVERSED (46,XX) MALES

Sex-reversed (46,XX) males are those phenotypic males who have bilateral testes. In 1971 de La Chapelle tabulated 45 cases,[120] and since then perhaps another 15 cases have been reported. 46,XX males with unstimulated yet normally differentiated male external genitalia usually have testes that are similar in size and histology to those of 47,XXY males. Both 46,XX males and 46,XX true hermaphrodites develop testes contrary to the assumption that an intact Y chromosome is necessary for testicular differentiation. Possible explanations include 1) undetected 46,XX/46,XY chimerism or 46,XX/47,XXY mosaicism, 2) loss of a Y-chromosome-containing cell line after initiation of testicular differentiation, 3) translocation of testes determinant(s) from the Y to the X, 4) translocation of testes determinant(s) from the Y to an autosome, and 5) a mutant gene.[2,121,122] The existence of several animal models[110] and several familial aggregates of human sex-reversal[121,122] support the last hypothesis,[2] but anomalous Xg distributions and other data suggest other possibilities in certain cases.

Apparently no 46,XX males have developed gonadal tumors or breast carcinoma. It is relevant that in sex-reversed (Sxr) mice germ cells are present in embryonic testes, although not present in the testes of adult animals.[110] Thus, not only are XX germ cells incapable of developing into spermatozoa, but they also direct stromal elements away from testicular differentiation. The lack of gonadal tumors in 46,XX human males or in 40,XX male mice indicates that XX germ cells may exist in the gonads of a phenotypic male without incurring an increased risk of neoplastic transformation.

FEMALE PSEUDOHERMAPHRODITISM

Genetic Forms

The genetic forms of female pseudohermaphroditism can be divided into those in which an adrenal biosynthetic error exists (adrenal hyperplasia) and those in which no such error exists.

Adrenal Hyperplasia. This condition results from deficiencies of various enzymes in adrenal and gonadal biosynthetic pathways: adrenal lipoid hyperplasia (deficiency of 20, 22-desmolase or 20 α-hydroxylase), 3β-ol dehydrogenase,

17α-hydroxylase, 21α-hydroxylase, 11β-hydroxylase, 17, 20-desmolase, and 17-ketosteroid reductase.[2,123] Adrenal lipoid hyperplasia, 3β-ol dehydrogenase deficiency, 21α-hydroxylase deficiency and 11β-hydroxylase deficiency cause female pseudohermaphroditism. 17α-hydroxylase deficiency is one cause of sexual infantilism in females and one cause of male pseudohermaphroditism. 17, 20-desmolase deficiency and 17-ketosteroid reductase deficiency can cause pseudohermaphroditism in males, but have not been reported in females.

The common pathogenesis for each type involves decreased production of glucocorticoids. In addition to its glucocorticoid properties, cortisol regulates ACTH secretion by negative feedback inhibition. If cortisol production is decreased, ACTH production is increased. Elevated ACTH levels lead to increased quantities of steroid precursors from which androgens are synthesized. The fetal adrenal begins to function during the 3rd month of embryonic development; thus, excess androgen production begins in utero and virilizes the external genitalia of female fetuses. Müllerian development and ovarian development are unaffected because neither are androgen-dependent.

Adrenal neoplasia has been reported, but appears to be rare in patients with adrenal hyperplasia, even if affected patients are not treated with cortisol during childhood. Thus, increased ACTH secretion does not predispose to neoplasia. Ovarian and genital tumors are also rarely associated, indicating that exposure in utero to excess androgens does not affect the potential for ovarian or genital carcinoma.

Other Genetic Forms. There are several nonadrenal genetic forms of female pseudohermaphroditism, but neoplasia has not been reported in any.[124] These rare syndromes are considered elsewhere.[2]

Teratogenic Forms. Female pseudohermaphroditism can result from administration of androgens or certain progestins to the pregnant female. If administered in an appropriate dose and at an appropriate time during embryonic development, female offspring may show 1) phallic enlargement, 2) labioscrotal fusion, 3) displacement of the urethral orifice from its normal site, and 4) failure of urogenital sinus invagination. Androgens and progestins capable of causing female pseudohermaphroditism include testosterone, 6α-methyl testosterone, ethisterone, norethindrone, and norethindrone acetate.[2,125] Teratogenic female pseudohermaphroditism may also result from a virilizing tumor in the mother.[126]

Neoplasia is apparently not increased in the teratogenic forms of female pseudohermaphroditism. This again indicates that exposure in utero to androgens predisposes neither to ovarian nor genital neoplasia, despite in utero hyperplasia of the external genitalia.

MALE PSEUDOHERMAPHRODITISM

Male pseudohermaphrodites are individuals with a Y chromosome whose external genitalia fail to develop as expected for normal males. Some investigators apply the term only to those individuals whose external genitalia are ambiguous enough to confuse the sex of rearing; however, for clinical purposes we prefer a broader definition.

Cytogenetic Forms: 45,X/46,XY and Variants

Individuals with both a 45,X cell line and at least one line containing a Y chromosome show a variety of phenotypes. The range extends from almost normal males with cryptorchidism or penile hypospadias to females indistinguishable from 45,X individuals who have the Turner stigmata.[72] The different phenotypes presumably reflect different tissue distributions of the various cell lines; however, this logical assumption is not proved. About half of 45,X/46,XY individuals have ambiguous external genitalia, hence 45,X/46,XY is best discussed in the context of male pseudohermaphroditism.

Individuals who are 45,X/46,XY may be grouped clinically into one of 3 categories, namely those with 1) unambiguous female external genitalia, usually associated with bilateral streak gonads, 2) ambiguous external genitalia, usually associated with either 2 dysgenetic testes or with one streak gonad and a contralateral dysgenetic testis, and 3) predominantly male external genitalia, usually associated with bilateral testes. Placement of a 45,X/46,XY patient into one of these 3 categories is not always possible. The etiology of 45,X/46,XY mosaicism is uncertain. Mitotic nondisjunction or anaphase lag are the usual explanations for mosaicism. However, the frequency with which structural rearrangements for the Y are associated suggests that the initial event might involve an intrachromosomal rearrangement, the monosomic line arising only secondarily.[127] This observation might be relevant to the question of neoplasia.

The incidence of neoplasia is definitely increased in 45,X/46,XY mosaicism, despite observations that the streak gonads of 45,X/46,XY patients are histologically indistinguishable from those of 45,X patients. Although it is clinically preferable to categorize 45,X/46,XY patients according to their genital status, it is more logical to discuss the risk of neoplasia according to gonadal status: 1) bilateral dysgenetic testes, 2) unilateral testis and contralateral streak gonad, and 3) bilateral streak gonads.

We can estimate the risk of neoplasia by several approaches. First, 45,X/46,XY mosaicism is so rare that until recently cases with neoplasia were probably no more likely to be reported than cases without neoplasia. In 1968, Pfeiffer et al[72] reviewed 79 cases. Four of the 23 cases (17.4%) with bilateral testes had a gonadoblastoma or dysgerminoma, all developing during the 2nd decade. Five of the 34 cases (14.7%) with a streak gonad and a contralateral testis had a tumor. None of the 22 cases with bilateral streak gonads had a tumor. Second, a relatively unbiased estimate of the risk of neoplasia might be obtained by analyzing patients routinely explored surgically. About 37 patients have been so explored; 5 (13%) had a tumor.[86,87,89,128–130] Thus, by either approach the prevalence of neoplasia seems to be about 15–20%, perhaps lower in patients with bilateral streak gonads or with nearly normal testes.

The prevalence of neoplasia, specifically gonadoblastomas and dysgerminomas, is, therefore, increased in both XY gonadal dysgenesis and in 45,X/46,XY mosaicism. Possible explanations were considered above: 1) the increased prevalence might reflect the existence of poorly differentiated XY gonadal tissue in an intraabdominal position, or 2) the particular process, genetic or cytogenetic, that produces 45,X/46,XY mosaicism might confer an increased propensity for neoplasia. That the risk is increased in both XY gonadal dysgenesis and 45,X/46,XY mosaicism suggests that the first hypothesis is correct. That Y-structural rearrangements are frequently associated with 45,X/46,XY[127] supports the second, inasmuch as a tendency to chromosomal breakage and rearrangement might lead to neoplastic clones. One as yet unproved unifying hypothesis might be that 45,X/46,XY mosaicism results from a somatic mutation that exerts its gonadal effect in a fashion similar to the mutant gene causing XY gonadal dysgenesis. Such a gene might lead to chromosomal nondisjunction (perhaps limited to germ cells, thus undetectable in XY gonadal dysgenesis), to anaphase lag, or to chromosomal breakage which secondarily gives rise to a monosomic (45,X) line.

The practical point is that all 45,X/46,XY or XY gonadal dysgenesis patients, possibly excepting nearly normal 45,X/46,XY males with scrotal testes, should be offered gonadal extirpation relatively soon after ascertainment, irrespective of age. Surgery is especially urgent if such a patient shows breast development because that sign usually signifies an estrogen-secreting tumor, namely a gonadoblastoma or a dysgerminoma.

GENETIC FORMS

Anomalies in Individuals with Abnormal yet Ambiguous Male Genitalia. In these patients the external genitalia are abnormal, yet not to the extent that the sex of rearing is questioned.

a) Hypospadias and Penile Anomalies. The incidence of gonadal or genital tumors is not increased in simple hypospadias, ie hypospadias associated with neither 45,X/46,XY mosaicism nor with one of the types of male pseudohermaphroditism to be discussed in later sections. However, many patients with hypospadias have testicular abnormalities, including cryptorchidism; thus, a slight increase in testicular neoplasia would not be surprising. In other penile anomalies — epispadias, micropenis, absence of the penis, diphallus — the incidence of neoplasia is apparently not increased.

b) Persistence of Müllerian Derivatives. Sometimes the uterus and fallopian tubes persist in otherwise normal males. The external genitalia, wolffian derivatives, and testes develop as expected for males; at puberty virilization occurs. There are 6 families with multiple affected sibs, and approximately 80 sporadic cases.[131] The disorder results from a mutant autosomal recessive gene.[131] Presumably the müllerian ducts fail to undergo the regression expected in males, an occurrence that could result either from end-organ insensitivity to the müllerian-inhibitory factor or from failure of the testes to elaborate the müllerian-inhibitory factor.

Testicular neoplasia has occurred in several affected individuals: seminomas,[131, 132] a choriocarcinoma,[133] an embryonal carcinoma,[134] teratomas,[135, 136] and a gonadoblastoma.[137] The frequency of testicular neoplasia may or may not be higher than the frequency in cryptorchid but otherwise normal males. Because germ cells are presumed to be originally normal in these patients, the occurrence of testicular neoplasia supports the concept that the intra-abdominal environment is oncogenic. On the other hand, one patient had a gonadoblastoma (Fig. 5),[137] a tumor present almost exclusively in patients with XY gonadal dysgenesis or 45,X/46,XY mosaicism. Thus, one might suspect an etiologic relationship between persistence of müllerian derivatives in males and either XY gonadal dysgenesis or 45,X/46,XY mosaicism. However, neither clinical nor genetic data support such a relationship. In fact, in the syndrome of persistent müllerian derivatives the chromosomal complement is normal and the testes are histologically normal except for features known to arise secondary to cryptorchidism. Moreover, no family has been reported in which one member had the syndrome of persistent müllerian derivatives and another member had 45,X/46,XY mosaicism.

Genital Anomalies Associated with Multiple Malformation Patterns. Simple hypospadias or genital ambiguity may occur in individuals with multiple malformation patterns. Because of the associated somatic anomalies a diagnosis is usually not difficult. A list of these syndromes has been tabulated elsewhere.[2]

One especially interesting syndrome[138, 139] is characterized by 1) male genital ambiguity, 2) the Wilms tumor, and 3) congenital nephrosis.

The renal disorder consists of 1) cystic dilatation of the proximal tubules and glomerular spaces, 2) glomerular changes ranging from immature glomeruli to hypercellular or solidified glomeruli, 3) thickening and degeneration of arteriolar walls, and 4) interstitial fibrosis. A given individual may have genital ambiguity, the Wilms tumor and congenital nephrosis, or he may have any 2 of the 3 features. It is tempting to postulate that a single mechanism — teratogenic or genetic — is responsible for the particular types of genital ambiguity, congenital nephrosis, and the Wilms tumor present in this syndrome. This situation is reminiscent of the postulated relationship between the Wilms tumor and aniridia.[105]

Male Pseudohermaphroditism Associated with a Demonstrable Enzyme Deficiency. Relatively few cases of male pseudohermaphroditism can be shown to result from an enzyme deficiency, although enzyme deficiencies probably often pass undetected. Deficiencies have been reported for 1) 20, 22-desmolase or 20α-hydroxylase (adrenal lipoid hyperplasia),[140] 2) 3β-ol dehydrogenase deficiency,[141] 3) 17α-hydroxylase deficiency,[142] 4) 17, 20-desmolase deficiency,[143] 5) 17-ketosteroid reductase deficiency,[144] and 6) 5α-reductase,[145,146] the enzyme that converts testosterone to dihydrotestosterone. All these disorders result in genital ambiguity in males; in none has neoplasia been reported.

Complete Testicular Feminization. In testicular feminization 46,XY individuals have bilateral testes (usually intraabdominal) (Fig. 8), female external genitalia, a blindly ending vagina, and no müllerian derivatives.[147] Breast development and puberal feminization occur as expected for normal females. The disorder results from androgen insensitivity, probably due to an abnormal cytosol receptor for androgen.[148] Complete testicular feminization is inherited as either an X-linked recessive or a male-limited autosomal dominant trait.

Despite puberal feminization some individuals with testicular feminization have clitoral enlargement and labioscrotal fusion. To these patients the term incomplete testicular feminization may be applied. We do not apply this term to androgen-insensitive patients who have slight clitoral hypertrophy but otherwise normal female genitalia. Both complete testicular feminization and incomplete testicular feminization are inherited similarly, but they are definitely distinct conditions.

The frequency of gonadal neoplasia is generally considered to be increased in complete testicular feminization, although etiology of the neoplasia remains uncertain. That is, does the risk of neoplasia merely reflect the increased risk incurred by any cryptorchid testes or is the risk a specific function of the mutant gene (Tfm) that causes testicular feminization?

In 1963, Morris and Mahesh reviewed 187 cases of testicular feminization.[147] Their sample comprised all cases reported up to that time. Eleven of the 50 cases (22%) over age 30 had a malignant tumor, usually a seminoma. Only 3 of the 127 cases under age 30 had a tumor — one patient in her 2nd decade, and 2 patients in their 3rd decade. However, many of these 187 cases were reported because of the associated neoplasia; thus, we can assume that these prevalence figures represent the maximal risk.

Most investigators agree with Morris and Mahesh that the risk of neoplasia is small prior to age 25–30.[73,124,149,150] For this reason most physicians prefer to leave the testes in situ until after puberal feminization. Thereafter, orchiectomy should probably be performed. The risk of neoplasia in older patients could be greater. In postpuberal patients benign tubular adenomas (Pick adenomas) are especially common, probably as result of increased secretion of LH, a characteristic of testicular feminization (see [2]). The precise risk of carcinomatous change is unknown, but it is probably less than the 22% estimated by Morris and Mahesh.[147] For example, Dewhurst[150] observed no cases of neoplasia in his sample, and malignancy is rarely detected in testicular feminization patients who

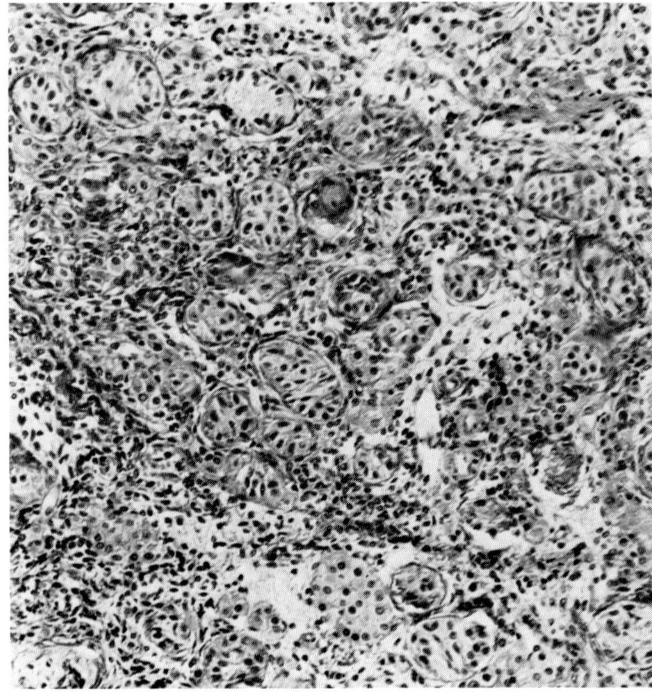

Fig. 8. Intraabdominal testis of a 39-year-old patient with testicular feminization. The tubules contain no lumens. Leydig cells are present in the stroma. No fibrosis or hyalinization is present (× 175).

are ascertained in surveys of patients with amenorrhea.[151–154] Thus, the incidence of carcinoma in older patients may be as high as about 20%, or it may be much lower. A reasonable estimate for the frequency of neoplastic transformation in Tfm might be 2–5%, a risk only slightly higher than the risk of neoplastic transformation in cryptorchid testes of otherwise normal men. Thus, carcinomatous transformation in Tfm may only be a function of the intraabdominal position of the testes, hence not necessarily related to the mutant gene per se. Supporting this thesis that carcinomatous degeneration occurs as result of some of the same factors that cause carcinomatous degeneration in cryptorchid testes are the similar spectrum of tumors and the similar ages of tumor onset in the 2 situations, namely the 3rd decade and later. Unlike the usual situation in cryptorchid men, however, we must assume that Tfm germ cells were originally normal, and the occurrence of neoplasia in Tfm supports the thesis that an intraabdominal environment predisposes to testicular neoplasia, irrespective of the cause of cryptorchidism.

The incidence of nongonadal neoplasia is apparently not increased in Tfm individuals. An analysis of nongonadal tumor prevalences in Tfm might, incidentally, distinguish between tumors that have a higher frequency in genetic males (46,XY) and tumors that only have a higher frequency in individuals with high androgen levels. If the former, but not the latter, were etiologically important, the incidence of a given tumor would be the same in normal males as in Tfm males; in both the incidence would be higher than in normal females (46, XX).

Incomplete Testicular Feminization. At puberty patients with incomplete testicular feminization display feminization as result of androgen insensitivity, yet their external genitalia are, nonetheless, characterized by phallic enlargement and partial labioscrotal fusion.[2, 155, 156] Both incomplete testicular feminization and complete testicular feminization share the following features: bilateral testes with similar histologic features, no müllerian derivatives, puberal breast development, lack of puberal virilization, and normal male plasma testosterone levels. The latter is important because certain patients with an error in testosterone biosynthesis (eg deficiency of 17α-hydroxylase) are phenotypically similar to those with incomplete testicular feminization. Markedly decreased testosterone levels usually exclude the latter. In incomplete testicular feminization, the incidence of gonadal neoplasia is, perhaps surprisingly, not increased. This may be related to the relatively high frequency with which affected individuals have inguinal or labial testes.

Reifenstein Syndrome. Most individuals said to have the Reifenstein syndrome[157] resemble incomplete testicular feminization. We only apply the appellation Reifenstein syndrome to androgen-sensitive males with small testes, a relatively normal phallus except for a proximally displaced urethral orifice, no vagina-like perineal orifice, a lack of puberal virilization, and elevated pituitary gonadotropin.[158, 159] Testes are usually located in the scrotum. This X-linked recessive or male-limited autosomal dominant syndrome must be differentiated from deficiencies of 17α-hydroxylase, 17, 20-desmolase, and 17-ketosteroid reductase. Neoplasia appears to be rare in patients with the Reifenstein syndrome.

Pseudovaginal Perineoscrotal Hypospadias (Possible 5α-Reductase Deficiency). Individuals with pseudovaginal perineoscrotal hypospadias (PPSH) have ambiguous external genitalia, but otherwise develop as expected for males. At puberty they undergo virilization — phallic enlargement, increased facial hair, muscular hypertrophy, voice deepening, and no breast development.[158, 159] Their testes are normal in size and usually scrotal or inguinal in location. Spermatogenesis may proceed into meiotic pachytene.[2, 160] PPSH, an autosomal recessive disorder, probably results from the deficiency of 5α-reductase,[145, 146] the enzyme that converts testosterone to dihydrotestosterone.

Testicular neoplasia has not been reported in PPSH individuals.

Anorchia: the Syndrome of Rudimentary Testes. Males with anorchia have unambiguous male external genitalia, normal wolffian derivatives, and no detectable gonadal tissue.[161] Some investigators prefer not to designate anorchic patients as male pseudohermaphrodites; however, because of their relationship to individuals with agonadia we believe that it is helpful clinically to consider anorchia as a form of male pseudohermaphroditism. Anorchia may result from torsion of the testicular arterial supply after the fetal testes elaborated those factors necessary for external genital masculination, wolffian differentiation, and müllerian inhibition.[161]

A related disorder is the syndrome of rudimentary testes, a designation applied to individuals with a small yet well-differentiated penis and very small testes (perhaps less than 1 cm in greatest diameter).[162, 163]

The frequency of neoplasia is apparently not increased in either of these disorders.

Agonadia. In agonadia the gonads are absent, the external genitalia are abnormal, and all but rudimentary müllerian or wolffian derivatives are absent. Somatic anomalies are often present. Affected sibs have been described,[164] but otherwise no etiologic factors have been identified. An explanation for this disorder must account not only for the absence of gonads but also for both abnormal external genitalia and the near absence of wolffian and müllerian derivatives. Possible explanations include 1) transient fetal testicular function that exists long enough to inhibit müllerian development yet not long enough to permit complete male genital development, or 2) an insult involving the entire gonadal, ductal, and genital system — either defective anlage, defective connective tissue, or a teratogen. Neoplasia has not occurred in any of the 10 reported cases.[164, 165]

CONCLUSIONS

In certain disorders of abnormal sexual differentiation the prevalence of neoplasia is higher than in normal individuals. The frequency varies among these disorders, and different etiologies may be responsible for the increased risks.

1. Four to 11% of males with testicular carcinoma have been cryptorchid. A cryptorchid testis is at least 14 times more likely to undergo neoplastic transformation than a normal scrotal testis. Moreover, the risk of neoplasia is decreased only if orchiopexy is performed prior to age 6–10 years. Neoplasia is probably a function of both the testes being in an intraabdominal environment and their being dysgenetic. If orchiopexy cannot be performed prior to age 6–10 years, orchiectomy should be considered if cryptorchidism is unilateral.

2. In those forms of gonadal dysgenesis not associated with a Y chromosome there is no increase in neoplasia, suggesting that elevated gonadotropin levels per se are not carcinogenic.

3. Gonadal tumors are found in 20–30% of individuals with XY gonadal dysgenesis; the tumors are almost exclusively gonadoblastomas or dysgerminomas, both of which usually arise in the 2nd or 3rd decade. Similar tumors are found in 15–20% of 45,X/46,XY individuals, also arising at a similar age. In both situations the neoplastic transformation could be a) secondary to the existence of XY gonadal tissue in an inhospitable position, or b) integrally related to the process – genetic or cytogenetic – that produces the dysgenetic gonads. The risk of neoplasia is sufficiently high that these patients should be offered gonadal extirpation shortly after diagnosis, except possibly for nearly normal males with scrotal testes.

4. The prevalence of gonadal tumors is not increased in the Klinefelter syndrome, again suggesting that gonadotropins are not carcinogenic per se. However, Klinefelter patients are 20 times more likely to develop carcinoma of the breast than 46,XY males.

5. In female pseudohermaphrodites there is apparently no increased risk of neoplasia, suggesting that neither increased ACTH levels nor in utero exposure to androgens are carcinogenic per se.

6. Neoplasia rarely arises in true hermaphrodites or 46,XX males.

7. Neoplasia occurs in complete testicular feminization but rarely in incomplete testicular feminization, the Reifenstein syndrome, pseudovaginal perineoscrotal hypospadias (PPSH), anorchia, agonadia, or syndromes characterized by errors in testosterone biosynthesis. In complete testicular feminization the risk of malignant tumors is small prior to age 25. After age 25 it is probably less than usually stated in the texts, and it may be no higher than 2–5%. However, orchiectomy should probably be performed after puberal feminization.

ACKNOWLEDGMENT

We wish to thank Dr. Robert Wahl for supplying us with Figures 2–4 and 6–8.

REFERENCES

1. Special Article: Classification and nomenclature of malformation. Lancet 1: 798, 1974.

2. Simpson, J. L: "Abnormal Sexual Development in Man." New York: Academic Press. (In press.)

3. Doll, R. Payne, P. and Waterhouse, J.: "Cancer Incidence in Five Continents. A Technical Report." Berlin: Springer-Verlag, 1966.

4. Janovski, N. A. and Paramanandhan, T. L.: "Ovarian Tumors: Tumors and Tumor-like Conditions of the Ovaries, Fallopian Tubes and Ligaments of the Uterus." Stuttgart: George Thieme, 1973.

5. Cramer, D. W. and Cutler, S. J.: Incidence and histopathology of malignancies of the female genital organs in the United States. Am. J. Obstet. Gynecol. 118: 443, 1974.

6. Fathalla, M. F.: Factors in the causation of ovarian carcinoma. Obstet. Gynecol. Surv. 27:751, 1972.

7. Lilienfeld, A. M., Levin, M. L. and Kessler, I. T.: "Cancer in the United States." Cambridge: Harvard University Press, 1972.

8. Julian, C. G.: Germinal epithelial neoplasia of the ovary. Clin. Obstet. Gynecol. 17:241, 1974.

9. Jimerson, G. K.: Germ cell tumors of the ovary. The role of pathology in diagnosis and management. Clin. Obstet. Gynecol. 17:229, 1974.

10. Novak, E. R. and Woodruff, J. D.: "Gynecologic and Obstetric Pathology," 7th Ed. Philadelphia: W. B. Saunders, 1974.

11. Scully, R. E.: Recent progress in ovarian cancer. Hum. Pathol. 1:73, 1970.

12. Fathalla, M. F.: Gonadal tumors in intersex patients. In Rashad, M. N. and Morton, W. R. M. (eds.): "Selected Topics on Genital Anomalies and Related Subjects." Springfield: Charles C Thomas, 1969.

13. Norris, H. J. and Jensen, R. D.: Relative frequency of ovarian neoplasms in children and adolescents. Cancer 30:713, 1972.

14. Norris, H. J. and Chorlton, I.: Functioning tumors of the ovary. Clin. Obstet. Gynecol. 17:189, 1974.

15. Teilum, G.: Classification of ovarian tumors. Acta Obstet. Gynecol. Scand. 31:292, 1952.

16. Bettinger, H. F.: Comments on homologous tumours of the ovary and testis. Acta Pathol. Microbiol. Scand. (A) (Suppl. 80) 233:15, 1972.

17. Malkasian, G. D., Jr. and Symmonds, R. E.: Treatment of unilateral and encapsulated ovarian dysgerminoma. Am. J. Obstet. Gynecol. 90:379, 1964.

18. Teilum, G.: "Special Tumors of Ovary and Testis. Comparative Pathology and Histologic Identification." Philadelphia: J. B. Lippincott, 1971.

19. Beilby, J. O. W. and Todd, P. J.: Yolk sac tumour of the ovary. J. Obstet. Gynecol. Br. Commonw. 81:90, 1974.

20. Gaillard, J. A.: Yolk-sac tumour patterns and entoblastic structures in polyembryomas. Acta Pathol. Microbiol. Scand. (A) (Suppl. 80) 233:18, 1972.

21. Huntington, R. W. and Bullock, W. K.: Endodermal sinus and other yolk sac tumours, a reappraisal. Acta Pathol. Microbiol. Scand. (A) (Suppl. 80) 233: 26, 1972.

22. Smith, J. P., Rutledge, F. and Sutow, W. W.: Malignant gynecologic tumors in children: Current approaches to treatment. Am. J. Obstet. Gynecol. 116:261, 1973.

23. Linder, D., McCaw, B. K. and Hecht, F.: Parthenogenic origin of benign ovarian teratomas. N. Engl. J. Med. 292:63, 1975.

24. Woodruff, J. D. and Jimerson, G. K.: Ovarian teratomata. Prog. Clin. Cancer 5:195, 1973.

25. Abell, M. R., Johnson, V. J. and Holtz, F.: Ovarian neoplasms in childhood and adolescence. Am. J. Obstet. Gynecol. 92:1059, 1965.

26. Scully, R. E.: Gonadoblastoma. Cancer 25:1340, 1970.

27. Teter, J.: Prognosis, malignancy, and curability of the germ-cell tumor occurring in dysgenetic gonads. Am. J. Obstet. Gynecol. 108:894, 1970.

28. Talerman, A.: Gonadoblastoma associated with embryonal carcinoma. Obstet. Gynecol. 43:138, 1974.

29. Scully, R. E.: Sex cord-mesenchyme tumours. In Gentil, F. and Junqueire, A. C. (eds.): "Ovarian Cancer," Berlin: Springer-Verlag, 1968, vol. II.

30. Smith, H. A. and Jones, T. C.: "Veterinary Pathology," 3rd Ed. Philadelphia: Lea and Febiger, 1966.

31. Fox, H., Agrawal, K. and Langley, F. A.: A clinicopathologic study of 92 cases of granulosa cell tumor of the ovary with special reference to the factors influencing prognosis. Cancer 35:231, 1975.

32. Goldston, W. R., Johnston, W. W., Fetter, B. F. et al: Clinicopathologic studies in feminizing tumors of the ovary. I. Some aspects of pathology and therapy of granulosa cell tumors. Am. J. Obstet. Gynecol. 112:422, 1972.

33. Pick., L.: Ueber Adenoma der männlichen und weiblichen Keimdrüse bei Hermaphroditismus verus und spurius. Berl. Klin. Wochenschr. 42:502, 1905.

34. Sternberg, W. H. and Roth, L. M.: Ovarian stromal tumors containing Leydig cells. I. Stromal-Leydig cell tumors and non-neoplastic cell transformation of ovarian stroma to Leydig cells. Cancer 32:940, 1973.

35. Novak, E. R., Kutchmeshgi, J., Mupas, R. S. and Woodruff, J. D.: Feminizing gonadal stromal tumors. Analysis of the granulosa-theca cell tumors of the ovarian tumor registry. Obstet. Gynecol. 38:701, 1971.

36. Bransilver, B. R., Ferenczy, A. and Richart, R. M.: Brenner tumors and Walthard cell nests. Arch. Pathol. 98:76, 1974.

37. Hagrimsson, J. and Scully, R. E.: Borderline and malignant Brenner tumors of the ovary. Acta Pathol. Microbiol. Scand. (A) (Suppl. 80) 233:56, 1972.

38. Jorgensen, E. O., Dockerty, M. B., Wilson, R. D. and Welch, J. S.: Clinicopathologic study of 53 cases of Brenner's tumors of the ovary. Am. J. Obstet. Gynecol. 108: 122, 1970.

39. Clarke, B. G.: The relative frequency and age incidence of principal urologic diseases. J. Urol. 98:701, 1967.

40. Mostofi, F. K.: Testicular tumors: Epidemiologic, etiologic, and pathologic features. Cancer 32:1186, 1973.

41. Koehler, P. R., Fabrikant, J. I. and Dickson, R. J.: Observations on the behavior of testicular tumors with comments on racial incidence. J. Urol. 87:577, 1962.

42. Sharma, K. C., Gaeta, J. F., Bross, I. D. et al: Testicular tumors. Histologic and epidemiologic assessment. N. Y. State J. Med. 72:2421, 1972.

43. Sherman, F. P., Ciavarra, V. A. and Cohen, M. J.: Testis tumors in negroes. Urology 2:318, 1973.

44. Boatman, D. L., Culp, D. A. and Wilson, V. B.: Testicular neoplasms in children. J. Urol. 109:315, 1973.

45. Henry, S. C., Walsh, P. C. and Rotner, M. B.: Choriocarcinoma of the testis. J. Urol. 112:105, 1974.

46. Giebink, G. S. and Ruymann, F. B.: Testicular tumors in childhood. Review and report of three cases. Am. J. Dis. Child. 127:433, 1974.

47. Mount, B. M., Huvos, A. G. and Whitmore, W. F.: Leydig cell tumors of testes, including cryptorchid testes. N. Y. State J. Med. 72:601, 1972.

48. Weitzner, S. and Gropp, A.: Sertoli cell tumor of testis in childhood. Am. J. Dis. Child. 128:541, 1974.

49. Scorer, C. G.: The descent of the testis. Am. J. Dis. Child. 39:605, 1964.

50. Levin, A. and Sherman, J. O.: The undescended testis. Surg. Gynecol. Obstet. 136:473, 1973.

51. Mininberg, D. T. and Nesrin, B.: Chromosomal abnormalities in undescended testes. Urology 1:98, 1973.

52. Vandemark, N. L. and Free, M. J.: Temperature effects. In Johnson, A. D., Gomes, W. R. and Vandemark, N. L. (eds.): "The Testis," New York: Academic Press, 1970, vol. III.

53. Charney, C. W. and Wolgin, W.: The management of cryptorchism. Surg. Gynecol. Obstet. 102:177, 1956.

54. Sohval, A. R.: Histopathology of cryptorchidism. Am. J. Med. 16:346, 1954.

55. Robinson, J. N. and Engle, E. T.: Some observations on cryptorchid testis. J. Urol. 71:726, 1954.

56. Sohval, A. R.: Testicular dysgenesis as an etiologic factor in cryptorchidism. J. Urol. 72:693, 1954.

57. Salle, B., Hedinger, C. and Nicole, R.: Significance of testicular biopsies in cryptorchidism in children. Acta Endocrinol. Scand. 58:67, 1968.

58. Myers, R. P. and Kelalis, P. P.: Cryptorchidism reassessed. Is there an optimal time for surgical correction? Mayo Clin. Proc. 48:94, 1973.

59. Kiesewetter, W. B., Schull, W. R. and Fetterman, G. H.: Histologic changes in the testis following anatomically successful orchidopexy. J. Pediatr. Surg. 4:59, 1969.

60. Scorer, C. G. and Farrington, G. H.: "Congenital Deformities of the Testis and Epididymis," London: Butterworth, 1971.

61. Dinner, M. and Spitz, L.: The relationship of testicular tumors to maldescent. S. Afr. Med. J. 48:45, 1974.

62. Gehring, G. G., Rodriquez, F. R. and Woodhead, D. M.: Malignant degeneration of cryptorchid testes following orchiopexy. J. Urol. 112:354, 1974.

63. Dow, J. A. and Mostofi, F. K.: Testicular tumors following orchiopexy. South Med. J. 60:193, 1967.

64. Sohval, A. R.: Testicular dysgenesis in relation to neoplasm of the testicle. J. Urol. 75:285, 1956.

65. Johnson, D. E., Woodhead, D. M., Pohl, D. P. and Robinson, J. R.: Cryptorchism and testicular tumorigenesis. Surgery 63:919, 1968.

66. Atkinson, P. M.: The effects of early experimental cryptorchidism and subsequent orchidopexy on the maturation of the guinea-pig testicle. Br. J. Surg. 60:253, 1974.

67. Simpson, J. L.: Gonadal dysgenesis and abnormalities of the human sex chromosomes: Current status of phenotypic-karyotypic correlations. In Bergsma, D. (ed.): "Hypogonadism," Birth Defects: Orig. Art. Ser., vol. XI, no. 4. Miami: Symposia Specialists for The National Foundation—March of Dimes, 1975, p. 23.

68. Simpson, J. L., Christakos, A. C., Horwith, M. I. et al: Gonadal dysgenesis in individuals with apparently normal chromosomal complements. In Bergsma, D. (ed.): Part X. "The Endocrine System," Birth Defects: Orig. Art. Ser., vol. VII, no. 6. Baltimore: Williams & Wilkins Co. for The National Foundation—March of Dimes, 1971, p. 215.

69. Wertelecki, W., Fraumeni, J. F., Jr. and Mulvihill, J. J.: Nongonadal neoplasia in Turner's syndrome. Cancer 26:485, 1970.

70. Cutler, B. S., Forbes, A. P., Ingersoll, F. M. and Scully, R. E.: Endometrial cancer after stilbestrol therapy in gonadal dysgenesis. N. Engl. J. Med. 287:628, 1972.

71. Wilkinson, J., Friedrich, E. G., Jr., Mattingly, R. F. et al: Turner's syndrome with endometrial adenocarcinoma and stilbestrol therapy. Obstet. Gynecol. 42:193, 1973.

72. Pfeiffer, R. A., Lambertz, B., Friederiszick, F. K. et al: Die nosologische Sellung des XO/XY-Mosaizimus. Arch. Gynaekol. 206:369, 1968.

73. Schellhas, H. F.: Malignant potential of the dysgenetic gonad. Obstet. Gynecol. 44: 298; 455, 1974.

74. Frasier, S. D., Bashore, R. A. and Mosier, H. G.: Gonadoblastoma associated with pure gonadal dysgenesis in monozygous twins. J. Pediatr. 64:740, 1974.

75. Brøgger, A. and Strand, A.: Contribution to the study of the so-called pure gonadal dysgenesis. Acta Endocrinol. (Kbh.) 48:490, 1965.

76. Cohen, M. M. and Shaw, M. W.: Two XY siblings with gonadal dysgenesis and a female phenotype. N. Engl. J. Med. 272:1083, 1965.

77. Sternberg, W. H., Barclay, D. L. and Kloepfer, H. W.: Familial XY gonadal dysgenesis. N. Engl. J. Med. 278:695, 1968.

78. Stanesco, V., Maximilian, C., Florea, I. and Ciovîrnache, M.: Trois soeurs avec dysgénésis gonadale pure et caryotype XY. Ann. Endocrinol. (Paris) 29:449, 1968.

79. Chemke, J., Carmichael, R., Stewart, J. M. et al: Familial XY gonadal dysgenesis. J. Med. Genet. 7:105, 1970.

80. Espiner, E. A., Veale, A. M. O., Sands, V. E. and Fitzgerald, P. H.: Familial syndrome of streak gonads and normal male karyotype in five phenotypic females. N. Engl. J. Med. 283:6, 1970.

81. Talerman, A.: Gonadoblastoma and dysgerminoma in two siblings with dysgenetic gonads. Obstet. Gynecol. 38:416, 1971.

82. Berger, R., Binoux, M., Chassan, E. and Lejeune, J.: Dysgénésie gonadique pure familiale. Ann. Endocrinol. (Paris) 33:35, 1972.

83. Boczkowski, K.: Sibship occurrence of XY gonadal dysgenesis with dysgerminoma. Am. J. Obstet. Gynecol. 113:952, 1972.

84. Campendonico, I., Venegas, E., Saito, E. et al: Sindrome de Swyer (disgenesia gonadal pura) y neoplasias gonadales en tres hermanas. Rev. Chil. Obstet. Gynecol. (Santiago) 38:155, 1973.

85. Simpson, J. L., Summitt, R. and German, J.: Unpublished data.

86. Greenblatt, R. B., Byrd, J. R., McDonough, P. G. and Mahesh, V. B.: The spectrum of gonadal dysgenesis. Am. J. Obstet. Gynecol. 98:151, 1967.

87. Andrews, J.: Streak gonads and the Y chromosome. J. Obstet. Gynecol. Br. Commonw. 78:448, 1971.

88. Sarto, G. E.: Cytogenetics of fifty patients with primary amenorrhea. Am. J. Obstet. Gynecol. 119:14, 1974.

89. German, J. and Simpson, J. L.: Unpublished data.

90. Mittwoch, U.: "Genetics of Sex Determination," New York: Academic Press, 1973.

91. Knudson, A. G., Jr., Strong, L. C. and Anderson, D. E.: Heredity and cancer in man. Prog. Med. Genet. 9:113, 1973.

92. Murkerjee, D., Bowen, J. M., Trujillo, J. M. and Cork, A.: Increased susceptibility of cells from cancer patients with XY-gonadal dysgenesis to Simian Papovavirus 40 transformation. Cancer Res. 32:1518, 1972.

93. Artzt, K. and Bennett, D.: A genetically caused embryonal ectodermal tumor in the mouse. J. Natl. Cancer Inst. 48:141, 1972.

94. Bennett, D., Goldberg, E., Dunn, L. C. and Boyse, E. A.: Serological detection of a cell-surface antigen specified by the T (Brachyury) mutant gene in the house mouse. Proc. Natl. Acad. Sci. USA 69:2076, 1972.

95. Artzt, K., Dubois, P., Bennett, D. et al: Surface antigens common to mouse cleavage embryos and primitive teratocarcinomas in culture. Proc. Natl. Acad. Sci. USA 70: 2988, 1973.

96. Artzt, K., Bennett, D. and Jacob, F.: Primitive teratocarcinoma cells express a differentiation antigen specified by a gene at the T-locus in the mouse. Proc. Natl. Acad. Sci. USA 71:811, 1974.

97. Becker, K. L.: Clinical and therapeutic experiences with Klinefelter's syndrome. Fertil. Steril. 23:568, 1972.

98. Simpson, J. L., Morillo-Cucci, G., Horwith, M. et al: Abnormalities of human sex chromosomes. VI. Monozygotic twins with the complement 48,XXXY. Humangenetik 22:301, 1974.

99. Zaleski, W. A., Houston, C. S., Pozsonyi, J. and Ying, K. L.: The XXXXY chromosomal anomaly: Report of three new cases and review of 30 cases from the literature. Can. Med. Assoc. J. 94:1143, 1966.

100. Gustavson, K.-H., Gamstrop, I. and Meurling, S.: Bilateral teratoma of testis in two brothers with 47,XXY Klinefelter's syndrome. Clin. Genet. 8:5, 1975.

101. Cuenca, C. R. and Becker, K. L.: Klinefelter's syndrome and cancer of the breast. Arch. Intern. Med. 121:159, 1968.

102. Harnden, D. G., Maclean, N. and Langlands, A. O.: Carcinoma of the breast and Klinefelter's syndrome. J. Med. Genet. 8:460, 1971.

103. Scheike, O., Visfeld, J. and Peterson, B.: Male breast cancer. III. Breast carcinoma in association with the Klinefelter syndrome. Acta Pathol. Microbiol. Scand. 81:352, 1973.

104. Hagen, C., McNeilly, A. S., Arroe, M. et al: Prolactin levels in gynecomastia related to Klinefelter's syndrome. Lancet 2:57, 1974.

105. Miller, R. W.: Relation between cancer and congenital defects in man. N. Engl. J. Med. 275:87, 1966.

106. Coley, G. M., Otis, R. D. and Clark, W. E, II: Multiple primary tumors including bilateral breast cancers in a man with Klinefelter's syndrome. Cancer 27:1476, 1971.

107. Murkerjee, D., Bowen, J. and Anderson, D. E.: Simian Papovavirus 40 transformation of cells from cancer patient with XY/XXY mosaic Klinefelter's syndrome. Cancer Res. 30:1769, 1970.

108. Rohde, R. A.: Klinefelter's syndrome with pulmonary disease and other disorders. Lancet 2:149, 1964.

109. Van Niekerk, W. A.: "True Hermaphroditism," Hagerstown: Harper and Row, 1974.

110. Cattanach, B. M., Pollard, C. E. and Hawkes, S. G.: Sex-reversed mice: XX and XO males. Cytogenetics 10:318, 1971.

111. Park, I. J., Pyeatte, J. C. and Jones, H. W., Jr.: Gonadoblastoma in a true hermaphrodite with 46,XY genotype. Obstet. Gynecol. 40:466, 1972.

112. Polano, O.: Ueber wahre Zwitterbildung beim Menschen. Z. Geburtsh. Gynaekol. 83:114, 1921.

113. Essenberg, J. M. and Feinberg, I. M.: A case of true hermaphroditism in man. West. J. Surg. 45:474, 1937.

114. Weed, J. C., Segaloff, A., Wiener, W. B. and Douglas, J. W.: True hermaphroditism. Endocrine studies in a case of ovotestis. J. Clin. Endocrinol. 7:741, 1947.

115. Bani, U.: Addome acuto de cristi ovarica torta sul peduncolo in ermafrodite vero. Polidinico (Prat.) 63:1238, 1956.

116. Stirling, W. C.: Abnormal sex development. Report of a unique case of true ambisexuality. Med. Ann. D. C. 28:559, 1959.

117. Botella-Llusiá, J.: Sobre un nuevo et case de hermafroditismo verdadero. Ann. Acad. Nac. Med. (Madrid) 127:261, 1960.

118. Vaughn, J. and Gonzalez-Angulo, A.: True hermaphrodite with ovarian tumor. J. Urol. 86:776, 1961.

119. Moriarty, J. D.: True hermaphroditism. Report of a case with mammary carcinoma. Am. J. Pathol. 20:799, 1944.

120. de La Chapelle, A.: Analytic review. Nature and origin of males with XX sex chromosomes. Am. J. Hum. Genet. 24:71, 1972.

121. Berger, R., Abonyi, D., Nodat, A. et al: Hermaphrodisme vrai et (Garcon XX) dans une fratrie. Rev. Europ. Études. Clin. Biol. 15:330, 1970.

122. Kasdan, R., Nankin, H. R., Troen, P. et al: Paternal transmission of maleness in XX human beings. N. Engl. J. Med. 288:539, 1973.

123. New, M. and Levine, L.: Congenital adrenal hyperplasia. Adv. Hum. Genet. 43:251, 1973.

124. Jones, H. W., Jr. and Scott, W. M.: "Hermaphroditism, Genital Anomalies, and Related Endocrine Disorders," 2nd Ed. Baltimore: Williams & Wilkins Co., 1971.

125. Wilkins, L.: Masculinization of female fetuses due to use of orally given progestins. JAMA 172:1028, 1960.

126. Brentnall, C. P.: A case of arrhenoblastoma complicating pregnancy. J. Obstet. Gynaecol. Br. Commonw. 52:235, 1945.

127. German, J.: Abnormalities of human sex chromosomes. V. A. unifying concept in relation to the gonadal dysgeneses. Clin. Genet. 1:15, 1970.

128. Morishima, A. and Grumbach, M. M.: The interrelationship of sex chromosome constitution and phenotype in the syndrome of gonadal dysgenesis and its variants. Ann. N. Y. Acad. Sci. 155:695, 1968.

129. Desjeux, J.-F., Gagnon, J., Leboeuf, G. et al: Huit observations de mosaique XO/XY, dont une XO/XYq- avec gonadoblastome. Union Med. Can. 98:1667, 1969.

130. Marquez-Monter, H., Armendares, S., Buentello, F. and Villegas, J.: Histopathologic study with cytogenetic correlation in 20 cases of gonadal dysgenesis. Am. J. Clin. Pathol. 57:449, 1972.

131. Brook, C. G. D., Wagner, H., Zachmann, M. et al: Familial occurrence of persistent Müllerian structures in otherwise normal males. Br. Med. J. 1:771, 1973.

132. Boulvin, R.: A propos de trois cas de pseudohermaphrodisme masculin interne chez l'homme. Ann. Chir. 18:1340, 1964.

133. Taub, J.: Malignant testis tumor, cryptorchidism and polyorchidism in a pseudohermaphrodite. J. Urol. 71:475, 1954.

134. Metcalfe, R. H.: Uterus masculinus: Complete tubular hermaphroditism with teratomatous enlargement of an undescended testicle. Br. J. Surg. 18:335, 1930.

135. Dvořak, R.: Ueber einen Fall von Pseudohermaphroditismus masculinus internus (tubularis). Virchow. Arch. (Pathol. Anat.) 251:616, 1924.

136. d'Arcy McCrea, E.: Tubular hermaphroditism with teratoma of the internal genitalia. Br. J. Surg. 18:91, 1930.

137. Morillo-Cucci, G. and German, J.: Males with a uterus and fallopian tubes, a rare disorder of sexual development. In "The Endocrine System," op. cit. p. 229.

138. Drash, A., Sherman, F., Hartmann, W. H. and Blizzard, R. M.: A syndrome of pseudohermaphroditism, Wilms' tumor, hypertension and degenerative renal disease. J. Pediatr. 76:585, 1970.

139. Barakat, A. Y., Papadopolou, Z. L., Chandra, R. S. et al: Pseudohermaphroditism, nephron disorder and Wilms' tumor: A unifying concept. Pediatrics 54:366, 1974.

140. Kirkland, R. T., Kirkland, J. L., Johnson, C. M. et al: Congenital lipoid adrenal hyperplasia in an eight-year-old phenotypic female. J. Clin. Endocrinol. 36:488, 1973.

141. Jänne, O., Perheentupo, J. and Vikho, R.: Plasma and urinary steroids in an eight-year-old boy with 3β-hydroxysteroid dehydrogenase deficiency. J. Clin. Endocrinol. 31:162, 1970.

142. New, M. I.: Male pseudohermaphroditism due to 17α-hydroxylase deficiency. J. Clin. Invest. 49:1930, 1970.

143. Zachmann, M., Vollmin, J. A., Hamilton, W. and Prader, A.: Steroid 17, 20-desmolase deficiency: A new cause of male pseudohermaphroditism. Clin. Endocrinol. 1:369, 1972.

144. Saez, J. M., de Peretti, E., Morera, A. M. et al: Familial male pseudohermaphroditism with gynecomastia due to testicular 17-ketosteroid reductase defect. I. Studies in vivo. J. Clin. Endocrinol. 32:604, 1971.

145. Imperato-McGinley, J., Guerrero, L., Gautier, T. and Peterson, R. E.: Steroid 5α-reductase deficiency in man: An inherited form of male pseudohermaphroditism. Science 186:1213, 1974.

146. Walsh, P. C., Madden, J. D., Harrod, M. J. et al: Familial incomplete male pseudo-hermaphroditism, Type 2. N. Engl. J. Med. 291:944, 1974.

147. Morris, J. M. and Mahesh, V. B.: Further observations on the syndrome, "testicular feminization." Am. J. Obstet. Gynecol. 87:731, 1963.

148. Bardin, C. W.: Androgen metabolism and mechanism of action in male pseudo-hermaphroditism: A study of testicular feminization. Recent Prog. Horm. Res. 19:65, 1973.

149. Hauser, G. D.: Testicular feminization. In Overzier, C. (ed.): "Intersexuality," London: Academic Press, 1963.

150. Dewhurst, C. J.: The XY female. Am. J. Obstet. Gynecol. 109:675, 1971.

151. Bjorø, K.: Primary amenorrhea. Acta Obstet. Gynecol. (Suppl. 4) 44:1–126, 1965.

152. Shearman, R. P.: A physiological approach to the differential diagnosis and treatment of primary amenorrhea. J. Obstet. Gynecol. Br. Commonw. 75:1101, 1968.

153. Lewis, A. C. W.: Chromosomal aspects of primary amenorrhea. Proc. R. Soc. Med. 63:21, 1970.

154. Kallio, H.: Cytogenetic and clinical study on 100 cases of primary amenorrhea. Acta Obstet. Gynecol. (Suppl. 24) 21:1, 1973.

155. Park, I. J. and Jones, H. W., Jr.: Familial male hermaphroditism with ambiguous external genitalia. Am. J. Obstet. Gynecol. 108:1197, 1970.

156. Wilson, J. D., Harrod, M. J., Goldstein, J. L. et al: Familial incomplete male pseudo-hermaphroditism, Type 1. N. Engl. J. Med. 290:1097, 1974.

157. Reifenstein, E. C., Jr.: Hereditary familial hypogonadism. Clin. Res. 3:86, 1947.

158. Simpson, J. L., New, M., Peterson, R. E. and German, J.: Pseudovaginal perineo-scrotal hypospadias (PPSH) in sibs. In "The Endocrine System," op. cit. p. 140.

159. Opitz, J. M., Simpson, J. L., Sarto, G. E. et al: Pseudovaginal perineoscrotal hypo-spadias. Clin. Genet. 3:1, 1972.

160. Simpson, J. L.: Unpublished data.

161. Simpson, J. L., Horwith, M., Morillo-Cucci, G. et al: Bilateral anorchia: Discordance in monozygotic twins. In "The Endocrine System," op. cit. p. 196.

162. Bergada, C., Cleveland, W. W., Jones, H. W. and Wilkins, L.: Variants of embryonic testicular dysgenesis: Bilateral anorchia and the syndrome of rudimentary testes. Acta Endocrinol. 40:521, 1962.

163. Najjar, S. S., Takla, R. J. and Nassar, V. H.: The syndrome of rudimentary testes: Occurrence in five siblings. J. Pediatr. 84:119, 1974.

164. Sarto, G. E. and Opitz, J. M.: The XY gonadal agenesis syndrome. J. Med. Genet. 10:288, 1973.

165. Parks, G. A., Dumars, K. W., Limback, G. A. et al: "True agonadism": A misnomer? J. Pediatr. 84:375, 1974.

Hereditary Aspects of Ovarian and Testicular Neoplasia

Joe Leigh Simpson, MD and Guy Photopulos, MD

The hereditary aspects of gonadal neoplasia are not well understood, although familial aggregates and epidemiologic data suggest that genetic factors are more important than generally appreciated. Our purpose is to review the genetics of gonadal tumors that arise in individuals with normal sexual differentiation. We shall review familial aggregates and attempt to determine whether familial cases differ clinically from nonfamilial cases. Elsewhere in this volume[1] we discussed the relationship between neoplasia and the disorders of abnormal sexual differentiation.

TESTICULAR NEOPLASIA

Testicular neoplasia occurs in about 2—2.5/100,000 males in the United States and Canada.[2] It is more common in whites than in blacks.[3−5] Ninety-four percent of testicular tumors arise from germ cells; almost all the remainder arise from gonadal stroma.[6] There are four types of germ cell tumors: seminoma, embryonal carcinoma, choriocarcinoma, and teratoma; their characteristics were summarized previously.[1] About 40% of germ cell tumors are mixed cell types.[6]

Cryptorchidism and Testicular Neoplasia

About 10% of males with testicular neoplasia are or have been cryptorchid.[1,6] The probability that a cryptorchid testis will undergo neoplastic transformation is about 14 times greater than that of a normally descended testis.[6] The risk of neoplasia decreases if orchiopexy is performed prior to age 6—10 years, but not if performed thereafter.[1,7−9] Possible explanation for these phenomena is considered elsewhere.[1]

Birth Defects: Original Article Series, Volume XII, Number 1, pages 51—60
© 1976 The National Foundation

Cryptorchidism in otherwise normal males may be heritable[10, 11]; thus, familial cryptorchidism might be associated with familial testicular neoplasia.

Familial Testicular Germ Cell Tumors

Eighteen familial aggregates of testicular neoplasia have been reported (Table 1).[12–29] The affected kindreds include 6 families in which neoplasia occurred in twins,[12–17] 9 families in which neoplasia occurred in non-twin sibs,[18–26] 2 families in which both a father and his son were affected,[27, 28] and one family in which a man and his nephew were affected.[29] In addition, Gustavson et al[30] observed bilateral teratomas in each of 2 non-twin sibs with 47,XXY Klinefelter syndrome.

In these kindreds each affected family member had a germ cell tumor. However, in about half the aggregates different types of tumors were present within a single family. For example, in several families one brother had a seminoma, whereas another had a teratoma. Assuming the familial aggregates were not merely coincidental, this suggests that the etiologic factors that cause one type of germ cell tumor can also cause another type. The tumor histology might, as a corollary, be governed by factors different from those that initiated the neoplastic transformation. The age of onset and the behavior of the tumors appeared to be similar in familial and in nonfamilial cases. The frequency of bilateral tumors is apparently not increased in familial cases.

Parental consanguinity has not been reported, although complete pedigrees were usually not obtained. Cytogenetic studies were usually not performed. The available genetic data are most consistent with polygenic or multifactorial inheritance, but a single mutant gene could occasionally be responsible for testicular carcinoma.

OVARIAN NEOPLASIA

The incidence of ovarian neoplasia is about 5–10/100,000 females.[31] Ninety percent of ovarian tumors arise from germinal epithelium; the remainder rise from germ cells or from stromal cells (sex cord-mesenchyme).[32] Clinical characteristics of germ cell tumors, stromal cell tumors, and some epithelial tumors were summarized elsewhere in this volume.[1] The common germinal epithelial tumors are discussed in standard gynecologic texts.

Epidemiologic Aspects

The epidemiologic aspects of ovarian neoplasia have not been well studied. For example, many studies fail to distinguish between the various types. Nonetheless, some interesting data are available, as reviewed by Fathalla.[33] The incidence of ovarian neoplasia varies among countries; it is lower in Japan than in most occidental countries.[31] However, first-generation Japanese living

in the United States have about the same tumor incidence as American caucasians[34,35]; thus, genetic factors must not be the sole explanation for the racial
differences. The incidence is higher in Ashkenazi Jews than in Sephardic Jews,[36]
higher in South African Bantu than in American whites or blacks,[37] and higher
in American caucasians than in American Indians.[38] Some investigators believe
that blacks have a relatively higher incidence of malignant teratomas, dysgerminomas, and mesenchymal mixed tumors,[39] although Scully[40] has questioned
this assertion. Ovarian neoplasia is also more common in higher socioeconomic
classes in Great Britain.[41]

Epithelial Tumors

Seven familial aggregates of probable epithelial tumors have been reported.[42–48]
The histology, when stated, was usually papillary serous or adenocarcinoma. In
most of these families individuals in 2 or more generations were affected; in
other families[47,48] only sibs were affected. The ovarian tumors arising in these
kindreds do not appear to differ clinically from sporadically arising tumors. In
one family, 3 teen-aged sibs were affected[48]; however, in all other cases the age
of onset was similar in both familial and nonfamilial cases. The frequency of bilaterality was also similar.

These data suggest that either 1) some ovarian adenocarcinomas result from
single mutant gene(s), in most families probably autosomal dominant or X-
linked dominant, 2) polygenic or multifactorial factors exist, or 3) various family
members were exposed to the same oncogenic agent. That the prevalence of
ovarian epithelial tumors differs among various species also supports the existence
of genetic factors. For example epithelial tumors are the most common ovarian
tumor in humans, canine species, and egg-laying domestic hens; granulosa cell
tumors are the most common ovarian tumors in most other species.[49] These
data suggest that germinal epithelial tumors, which arise from the mesothelial
surface of the ovary, are more frequent in species in which the ovarian surface
epithelium is frequently disrupted by ovulation, without quiescent intervals.[33]

No familial aggregates of Brenner tumors or endometrioid tumors have been
reported. Finally, Lynch and Krush[50] have reported kindreds in which many
members either had carcinoma of the breast or epithelial carcinoma of the ovary.

Germ Cell Tumors

Ovarian germ cell tumors include teratomas, embryonal carcinomas (yolk
sac tumor, endodermal sinus tumor), dysgerminomas, gonadoblastomas, and
choriocarcinomas. Gonadoblastomas, discussed in our accompanying article,[1]
occur almost exclusively in 46,XY or 45,X/46,XY individuals. No familial aggregates of embryonal carcinoma have been reported.

Teratomas. Teratomas (dermoid tumors) may arise in gonadal or in extragonadal sites.[51,52] Nongonadal tumors, familial aggregates of which have been

TABLE 1. Summary of Clinical Data Derived From 17 Families in Which Multiple Members Had Testicular Neoplasia

Investigators	Relation	Age at Which Neoplasia Was Detected	Histologic Type	Cryptorchidism
Twins				
Champlin[12]		24	Embryonal	−
	Co-twin	31	Sarcoma	−
Domrich[13]		35	Embryonal	+
	Co-twin	39	Embryonal	+
Wells[14]	Co-twin		Seminoma	
			Seminoma	
Salm & Adlington[15]		40	Seminoma	+
	Co-twin	44	Seminoma	+
Stewart & Bagshaw[16]		37	Embryonal	−
	Co-twin	37	Seminoma	−
Villani[17]		24	Teratoma	+
	Co-twin	24	Teratocarcinoma	+
Non-twin Sibs				
Raven[18]		19	Not stated	
	Brother	38	Seminoma	
Lownes and Leberman[19]		32	Seminoma	
	Brother	53	Teratoma	
Willis[20]		38	Seminoma	+
	Brother	31	Teratoma	−
	Grandfather (?)	50	Not stated	−

Report	Relationship	Age	Histology
Hutter et al[21]		32	Embryonal/teratoma
	Brother	31	Seminoma
Beltrami & Luppi[22]		36	Retroperitoneal choriocarcinoma
	Brother	44	Embryonal carcinoma
Nordholt[23]		37	Teratoid
	Brother	26	
Myers & Mac-Pherson[24]		20	Teratocarcinoma
	Brother	25	Embryonal/Teratoma
Young & Bohne[25]		37	Seminoma
	Brother	45	Seminoma
Gulley et al[26]		31	Embryonal
	Brother	27	Seminoma
	Brother	34	Embryonal/seminoma
	Brother	40	Not studied
Father-Son Silber et al[27]		38	Seminoma
	Son	19	Teratocarcinoma
Arcadi[28]		51	Seminoma
	Son	28	Seminoma
Uncle-Nephew Vilček[21]		4	Teratocarcinoma
	Uncle	29	Seminoma

All cases involved germ cell tumors. + indicates presence; − absence; blank space no information. The tumors occurring in familial aggregates were similar in appearance, age of onset, and behavior to non-familial germ cell tumors. The father reported by Arcadi was obese; his son was possibly infertile.

reported,[51] may be related to sequestration of embryonic cells prior to differentiation and subsequent inhibition of their totipotential capacity.[52] By contrast, gonadal teratomas probably arise by parthenogenesis.[53]

Heritable tendencies in the etiology of ovarian dermoid tumors are suggested by 1) the relatively high prevalence of bilateral tumors, and 2) the relatively young age of onset — one half of all childhood ovarian tumors are dermoid tumors.[54] Bilaterality and early age of onset are characteristics of hereditary tumors.[55] Ovarian teratomas have been described in sisters,[56,57] in a mother and her 2 daughters,[49] in each of twins,[58] and in each of triplets.[59]

46,XX Dysgerminomas. Familial dysgerminomas may occur in individuals with XY gonadal dysgenesis or 45,X/46,XY mosaicism.[60] Familial aggregates rarely occur among 46,XX individuals, although Jackson reported dysgerminomas in 2 and perhaps 3 generations of a Jamaican kindred.[61]

Gonadoblastomas and 46,XY Dysgerminomas. Gonadoblastomas, and less often dysgerminomas, are the tumors that usually arise in individuals with XY gonadal dysgenesis or 45,X/46,XY mosaicism. These disorders are discussed in our previous article.[1]

Sex Cord-Mesenchyme

These tumors include granulosa cell tumors, theca cell tumors, Sertoli cell tumors, and Leydig cell tumors. Mixed varieties are common. Their clinical and histologic characteristics have been previously summarized.[1]

Granulosa Cell Tumors. In pure granulosa cell tumors the mean age is 50 years, yet the tumor may occur before puberty.[62] Familial aggregates of granulosa cell tumors are rare in otherwise normal females. However, ovarian tumors, principally granulosa cell tumors, are frequently associated with the Peutz-Jeghers syndrome.[63] In one series 16 of 115 patients with the Peutz-Jeghers syndrome had an ovarian tumor.[63]

Interestingly, granulosa cell tumors are the most common spontaneous ovarian tumor in many animals. In addition, granulosa cell tumors can be induced in rodents by irradiation, 9:10-dimethyl-1:2-benzanthracene, or progestational steroids[33,64]; tumor susceptibility depends upon the genotype of the animal.[65] The origin of granulosa cell tumors appears to be related to elimination of oogonia[33]; if no oogonia are present, granulosa cells might proliferate in response to increased pituitary gonadotropin.

Sertoli-Leydig Cell Tumors (Arrhenoblastomas). Reported familial aggregates of arrhenoblastomas include affected sibs,[66,67] an affected mother and her daughter,[68] and affected cousins.[69] Murad et al[70] also reported a family in which a 15-year-old girl, her maternal aunt, and her maternal grandmother each developed a virilizing ovarian tumor in their second decade. Histologic and electron microscopic studies indicated that the tumor in the 15-year-old girl consisted of both Sertoli and Leydig cells (arrhenoblastoma).

Fibromas and Fibrosarcomas

Ovarian fibrosarcomas, frequently associated with the basal cell nevus syndrome[71] and with neurofibromatosis (von Recklinghausen syndrome), were described in each of dizygotic twins,[72] but no other familial aggregates have been reported.

CONCLUSIONS

Genetic factors are probably more important in the etiology of gonadal neoplasia than generally appreciated.

Seventeen familial aggregates of testicular germ cell tumors have been reported. These include concordantly affected twins, affected sibs of non-consanguineous parents, and affected individuals in more than one generation. In a given family, affected members often had tumors of different histology, suggesting that the factors that cause one type of germ cell tumor may be the same as those that cause another type. Such an hypothesis is consistent with observations that many testicular germ cell tumors contain more than one cell type.

Several familial aggregates of ovarian tumors have been reported. Germinal epithelial tumors have been reported in multiple sibs as well as in individuals in more than one generation. The genetic data suggest that either 1) some ovarian epithelial tumors result from a mutant gene(s), probably autosomal dominant or X-linked dominant, or 2) polygenic or multifactorial factors play a role in the etiology of ovarian epithelial neoplasia. A few familial aggregates of teratomas (dermoid tumors), a germ cell tumor, have also been reported. The relatively high frequency of bilaterality and the relatively young age of onset also suggest that hereditary factors are important in teratomas. Familial aggregates of sex cord-mesenchyme tumors have also been reported. Granulosa cell tumors and certain other ovarian tumors are often associated with the Peutz-Jeghers syndrome.

REFERENCES

1. Simpson, J. L. and Photopulos, G.: The relationship of neoplasia to disorders of abnormal sexual differentiation. This volume.
2. Clarke, B. G.: The relative frequency and age incidence of principal urologic diseases. J. Urol. 98:701, 1967.
3. Koehler, P. R., Fabrikant, J. I. and Dickson, R. J.: Observations on the behavior of testicular tumors with comments on racial incidence. J. Urol. 87:577, 1962.
4. Sharma, K. C., Gaeto, J. F., Bross, I. D. et al: Testicular tumors. Histologic and epidemiologic assessment. N. Y. State J. Med. 72:2421, 1972.
5. Sherman, F. P., Ciavarra, V. A. and Cohen, M. J.: Testis tumors in Negroes. Urology 2:318, 1973.

6. Mostofi, F. K.: Testicular tumors: Epidemiologic, etiologic, and pathologic features. Cancer 32:1186, 1973.

7. Dinner, M. and Spitz, L.: The relationship of testicular tumors to maldescent. S. Afr. Med. J. 48:45, 1974.

8. Gehring, G. G., Rodriquez, F. R. and Woodhead, D. M.: Malignant degeneration of cryptorchid testes following orchiopexy. J. Urol. 112:354, 1974.

9. Dow, J. A., Oteen, N. C. and Mostofi, F. K.: Testicular tumors following orchiopexy. South. Med. J. 60:193, 1967.

10. Corbus, B. C. and O'Connor, V. J.: The familial occurrence of undescended testes. Report of six brothers with testicular anomalies. Surg. Gynecol. Obstet. 34:237, 1922.

11. Perrett, L. J. and O'Rourke, D. A.: Hereditary cryptorchidism. Med. J. Aust. 1:1289, 1969.

12. Champlin, H. W.: Similar tumors of testis occurring in identical twins. JAMA 95:96, 1930.

13. Domrich, H.: Über Leistenhodencarcinom bei Zwillingen. Arch. Klin. Chir. 197:848, 1940.

14. Wells, H. G.: Personal communication to Twinem, 1937. Cited by Macklin, M. T.: Analysis of tumors in monozygous and dizygous twins, with report of 15 unpublished cases. J. Hered. 31:277, 1940.

15. Salm, R. and Adlington, S. R.: Seminoma in identical twins. Br. J. Med. 2:964, 1962.

16. Stewart, J. R. and Bagshaw, M. A.: Malignant testicular tumors appearing simultaneously in identical twins: A case report. Cancer 18:895, 1965.

17. Villani, U.: Tumore concordante del testicolo in una coppia di gemelli morozigoti. Acta Genet. Med. Gemellol. 16:172, 1967.

18. Raven, R. W.: Tumours of the testis in two brothers. Lancet 2:870, 1934.

19. Lownes, J. B. and Leberman, P.: Tumors of the testis in brothers. Urol. Cutan. Rev. 43:205, 1939.

20. Willis, R. A.: "Pathology of Tumours," 2nd Ed. London: Butterworth & Co., Ltd., 1953.

21. Hutter, A. M., Jr., Lynch, J. L. and Schnider, B. I.: Malignant testicular tumors in brothers: A case report. JAMA 199:1009, 1967.

22. Beltrami, C. A. and Luppi, L. A.: Familiarita di tumori a cellule germinali. Riv. Pat. Clin. Sper. 9:267, 1968.

23. Nordholt, A. E.: Testitumoren bij broers bijn gelijktijdig tot maligne groei gekomen. Ned. Tijdschr Geneeskd. 115:1046, 1971.

24. Myers, G. H. and MacPherson, B. R.: Histologically similar testicular neoplasms occurring in brothers. J. Urol. 108:757, 1972.

25. Young, J. A. and Bohne, A. W.: Seminoma in non-twin brothers: A case report. J. Urol. 107:1000, 1972.

26. Gulley, I. M., Kowalski, R. and Neuhoff, C. F.: Familial occurrence of testicular neoplasms: A case report. J. Urol. 112:620, 1974.

27. Silber, S. J., Cittan, S. and Friedlander, G.: Testicular neoplasm in father and son. J. Urol. 108:889, 1972.

28. Arcadi, J. A.: Testicular neoplasms in father and son. J. Urol. 110:306, 1973.

29. Vilček, E.: Familiárny výskyt malígnych nádorov testis. Bratisl. Lek. Listy. 59:199, 1973.

30. Gustavson, K.-M., Gamstrop, I. and Meurling, S.: Bilateral teratoma of testis in two brothers with 47, XXY Klinefelter's syndrome. Clin. Genet. 8:5, 1975.

31. Doll, R., Payne, P. and Waterhouse, J.: "Cancer Incidence in Five Continents. A Technical Report." Berlin: Springer-Verlag, 1966.

32. Lilienfeld, A. M., Levin, M. L. and Kessler, I. I.: "Cancer in the United States." Cambridge: Harvard University Press, 1972.

33. Fathalla, M. F.: Factors in the causation and incidence of ovarian cancer. Obstet. Gynecol. Surv. 27:751, 1972.

34. Buell, P. and Dunn, J., Jr.: Cancer mortality among Japanese Issei and Nisei of California. Cancer 18:656, 1965.

35. Haenszel, W. and Kurihara, M.: Studies of Japanese migrants. 1. Mortality from cancer and other diseases among Japanese in the United States. J. Natl. Cancer Inst. 40:43, 1968.

36. Steinitz, R.: The Israel Cancer Registry. New cases of malignant neoplasms in 1960 and 1961. Ministry of Health, 1963. Cited in Kmet, J.: The role of migrant populations in studies of selected cancer sites: A review. J. Chronic. Dis. 23:305, 1970.

37. Higginson, J. and Oettlé, A. G.: Cancer incidence in the Bantu and "Cape colored" races of South Africa: Report of a cancer survey in the Transvaal (1953–1955). J. Natl. Cancer Inst. 24:589, 1960.

38. Smith, R. L.: Recorded and expected mortality among the Indians of the United States with special reference to cancer. J. Natl. Cancer Inst. 3:385, 1957.

39. Berg, J. W. and Baylor, S. M.: The epidemiologic pathology of ovarian cancer. Hum. Pathol. 4:537, 1973.

40. Scully, R. E.: The need for uniform terminology. Hum. Pathol. 4:602, 1973.

41. Registrar General of England and Wales. The Registrar General Decennial Supplement, England and Wales, 1931. Occupational Mortality. His Majesty's Stationary Office, London, 1938.

42. Lynch, F. W.: A clinical review of 110 cases of ovarian cancer. Am. J. Obstet. Gynecol. 32:753, 1936.

43. Liber, A. F.: Ovarian cancer in mother and four daughters. Arch. Pathol. 49:280, 1950.

44. Graham, J. B., Graham, R. M. and Scheuller, E. F.: Preclinical detection of ovarian cancer. Cancer 17:1414, 1964.

45. Lewis, A. C. W. and Davison, B. C. C.: Familial ovarian cancer. Lancet 2:235, 1969.

46. Li, F. P., Rappaport, A. H., Fraumeni, J. F. and Jensen, R. D.: Familial ovarian carcinoma. JAMA 214:1559, 1970.

47. Molloy, W. B.: Identical ovarian malignant disease in two sisters. Aust. N. Z. J. Obstet. Gynecol. 10:256, 1970.

48. McCrann, D. J., Jr., Marchant, D. J. and Bardawil, W. A.: Ovarian carcinoma in three teen-age siblings. Obstet. Gynecol. 43:132, 1974.

49. Smith, H. A. and Jones, T. C.: "Veterinary Pathology," 3rd. Ed. Philadelphia: Lea and Febiger, 1966.

50. Lynch, H. T. and Krush, A. J.: Carcinoma of the breast and ovary in three families. Surg. Gynecol. Obstet. 133:644, 1971.

51. Plattner, G. and Oxorn, H.: Familial incidence of ovarian dermoid cysts. Can. Med. Assoc. J. 108:892, 1973.

52. Ashley, D. J. B.: Origin of teratomas. Cancer 32:390, 1973.

53. Linder, D., McCaw, B. K. and Hecht, F.: Parthenogenic origin of benign ovarian teratomas. N. Engl. J. Med. 292:63, 1975.

54. Novak, E. R. and Woodruff, J. D.: "Gynecologic and Obstetric Pathology," 7th Ed. Philadelphia: W. B. Saunders, 1974.

55. Knudson, A. G., Jr., Strong, L. C. and Anderson, D. E.: Heredity and cancer in man. Prog. Med. Genet. 9:113, 1973.

56. Hollander, H. and Masterson, J. G.: Familial cystic teratoma of the ovary. Tex. Rep. Biol. Med. 25:483, 1967.

57. Sippel, A.: Dermoid of ovary in three sisters. Zentralbl. Gynaekol. 48:85, 1924.

58. Schauffler, G.: "Pediatric Gynecology." Chicago: Year Book Publishers, 1958.

59. Feld, D., Lalies, J. and Nathanson, M.: Bilateral ovarian dermoid cysts in triplets. Obstet. Gynecol. 33:324, 1969.

60. Scully, R. E.: Gonadoblastoma. Cancer 25:1340, 1970.

61. Jackson, S. M.: Ovarian dysgerminoma in three generations. J. Med. Genet. 4:112, 1967.

62. Fox, H., Agrawal, K. and Langley, F. A.: A clinicopathologic study of 92 cases of granulosa cell tumor of the ovary with special reference to the factors influencing prognosis. Cancer 35:231, 1975.

63. Dozois, R. R., Kemper, R. D. and Dahlin, D. C.: Ovarian tumors associated with the Peutz-Jeghers syndrome. Ann. Surg. 172:233, 1970.

64. Krarup, T.: Effect of 9, 10 dimethyl-1, 2-benzanthracene on the mouse ovary. Ovarian tumorigenesis. Br. J. Cancer 24:168, 1970.

65. Marchant, J.: Influence of the strain of ovarian grafts on the induction of breast and ovarian tumors in F1 NB C57B1 X1F hybrid mice by 9:10-dimethyl-1:2-benzanthracene. Br. J. Cancer 13:306, 1959.

66. Accado, M. and Condorelli, B.: Arrhenoblastoma in due Sorrelle. Riv. Pat. Clin. Sper. 7:171, 1966.

67. Serban, A. M. D., Coivirnache, M. and Maximilian, C.: Arrhenoblastome familial. Rev. Roum. Embryol. Cytol. Ser. Embryol. 5:11, 1968.

68. Javert, C. T. and Finn, W. F.: Arrhenoblastoma. The incidence of malignancy and the relationship to pregnancy, to sterility and to treatment. Cancer 4:60, 1951.

69. Goldstein, D. P. and Lamb, E. J.: Arrhenoblastoma in first cousins. Report of 2 cases. Obstet. Gynecol. 35:444, 1970.

70. Murad, T. M., Mancini, R. and George, J.: Ultrastructure of a virilizing ovarian Sertoli-Leydig cell tumor with familial incidence. Cancer 34:1440, 1973.

71. Clendenning, W. E., Herdit, J. R. and Block, J. B.: Ovarian fibromas and mesenteric cysts: Their association with hereditary basal cell cancer of the skin. Am. J. Obstet. Gynecol. 87:1008, 1963.

72. Macklin, M. T.: Tumors in monozygous and dizygous twins. Can. Med. Assoc. J. 44:604, 1941.

Cancer and Immunodeficiency Diseases

Charles H. Kirkpatrick, MD

The notion that the immune system provided a mechanism for early recognition and elimination of neoplastic cells was introduced by Thomas in 1959.[1] The proposal was extended by Burnet,[2] who suggested that the occurrence of malignant cells was a common event, but under normal circumstances the abnormal cells were destroyed by immunologic surveillance mechanisms of the host. Implicit in these proposals were two assumptions: 1) tumor cells must possess unique surface antigens that permit them to be recognized as foreign; and 2) the host must be capable of developing an appropriate and effective immune response against these antigens. A corollary to the second assumption predicted that cancer would occur more frequently in patients or animals with deficient immune responses.

During recent years substantial evidence has accumulated in support of both assumptions. Tumors induced by viruses or by chemical carcinogens have been shown to possess tumor-specific transplantation antigens.[3−8] Tumors induced by chemicals such as methylcholanthrene generally possess antigens specific for each tumor.[5−7] Thus, tumors induced by the same chemical, but occurring in different sites in the same animal or histologically similar tumors arising in the same tissues of syngenic animals usually have unique tumor antigens. In contrast, tumors produced by the same virus have similar antigens regardless of the location or histologic characteristics of the tumor.[3,4,7] The antigens of virus-induced tumors fall into two general categories. One group, exemplified by certain RNA viruses, continually sheds virus particles from the cell membranes, and the tumor antigens are similar to structural antigens of the virus. The second group is usually observed with certain DNA viruses; in these tumors the membrane-associated tumor antigens are not present either in the virus or in the host's cells prior to neoplastic transformation.[3]

Birth Defects: Original Article Series, Volume XII, Number 1, **pages 61−78**
© **1976 The National Foundation**

Antigens that are apparently tumor-specific have been demonstrated in a variety of human tumors including acute leukemia,[9] osteogenic sarcoma,[10,11] malignant melanoma,[12-14] the Burkitt tumor,[15] hepatoma,[16] neuroblastoma,[17] and gastrointestinal neoplasms.[18] Moreover, cell-mediated immune responses to tumor antigens have been demonstrated by both in vivo and in vitro techniques. Intradermal injections of tumor extracts into animals or tumor-bearing patients often produce typical delayed hypersensitivity responses.[14,15,19] Exposure of lymphocytes from tumor-bearing subjects to tumor extracts in vitro has induced lymphocyte transformation[19-22] and lymphokine production.[23-26] In other experiments, lymphocytes from cancer patients have shown specific cytotoxic activities against tumor cells.[11,17,27]

A role for cellular immunity in resistance to neoplasia has been suggested by experiments in which lymphoid cells from immune donors, when transferred to tumor-bearing animals or patients, caused either retardation of tumor growth or regression of tumor masses.[28-30] Moreover, application of chlorodinitrobenzene (CDNB) to cutaneous cancers in previously sensitized subjects has produced tumor regression through nonspecific effects of the cell-mediated immunologic inflammatory responses.[31] Currently, activation of the immune system with agents such as BCG is being investigated in tumor immunotherapy.[32,33]

Tumor-bearing animals and patients often have tumor-specific antibodies in their serum.[12,17] These antibodies indicate sensitization to tumor antigens, but their role in the pathogenesis of tumor growth is unclear. Under some conditions, antibodies clearly enhance tumor growth in vivo and block lymphocyte-mediated injury to tumor cells in vitro.[14,27,34]

In considering the interrelationships between the immune system and neoplasia, several possibilities must be considered: 1) Immunodeficiency syndromes render the host susceptible to infection with oncogenic agents; 2) deficiency diseases impair the ability of the host to destroy malignant cells that arise spontaneously; 3) oncogenic agents including chemicals and viruses may also have immunosuppressive properties that facilitate or enhance their oncogenic potential [35,36]; and/or 4) the neoplastic process itself may suppress the immune response and perpetuate tumor growth. In addition, one must consider the genetic and environmental factors that may predispose a potentially susceptible subject to development of neoplasia.

THE DEVELOPMENT OF THE IMMUNE SYSTEM AND ITS RELATIONSHIP TO THE PATHOGENESIS OF IMMUNE DEFICIENCY SYNDROMES

In some respects the study of the immune deficiency syndromes began in 1952 when Bruton discovered that a patient with recurrent infections was deficient in serum gamma globulin.[37] Other similar cases were soon recognized and by 1954 certain morphologic counterparts of this disease, such as the absence of plasma cells and germinal centers in lymphoid organs, were known. During the 1960s, experiments with immunologically manipulated chickens led to the formulation of the two-component model for the development of the immune system.[38] This model defined the relative independence of the cellular and humoral immune responses and provided explanations for the pathogenesis of certain congenital immunodeficiency diseases.

As shown in Figure 1, the source of potentially immunocompetent cells in postnatal animals is the bone marrow. In chickens, marrow-derived stem cells may receive differentiative influences from one of 2 sources, the thymus and the bursa of Fabricius, a lymphoid organ in the hindgut. An analogous organ has not been conclusively demonstrated in mammals, although Cooper and Lawton[39] have suggested that it may be the follicular areas of the gut-associated lymphoid tissues.

The bursa directs differentiation of cells that participate in antibody synthesis, and maturation of antibody-forming cells from stem cells is probably a two-step process.[40] The first phase occurs during embryonic life and is characterized by the formation of B lymphocytes, the precursors of antibody-forming cells. B cells are able to synthesize immunoglobulins and may be identified by the immunoglobulins on the cell membrane, as well as membrane receptors for aggregated immunoglobulin (IgG) and the third component (EAC).[41] The first B cells that appear in the embryo bear IgM and it has been postulated that these cells are the precursors of IgG- and IgA-bearing cells.[40] Differentiation and replication of B cells from stem cells does not require antigenic stimulation.

The second phase involves maturation of B cells into antibody-secreting cells, such as plasma cells. This step occurs in response to antigenic stimulation and involves only the subpopulation of B cells that are able to respond to that antigen. For many antigens, optimal antibody responses require cooperation by thymus-derived T lymphocytes and macrophages.[42, 43]

In vitro stimulation of normal B lymphocytes with pokeweed mitogen (PWM) causes them to release newly synthesized immunoglobulins into the cytoplasm and the culture media.[44] This phenomenon, described in more detail below, has been used to study the differentiative potential of lymphocytes of patients with a variety of hypogammaglobulinemic syndromes.

The second major pathway of lymphocyte differentiation involves maturation of stem cells into thymus-derived T lymphocytes and the effector cells of cell-mediated immunity. This process, too, is probably a two-stage event. The first stage involves formation of T cells that may be identified by their ability to spontaneously form rosettes with sheep erythrocytes.[41] Like the first

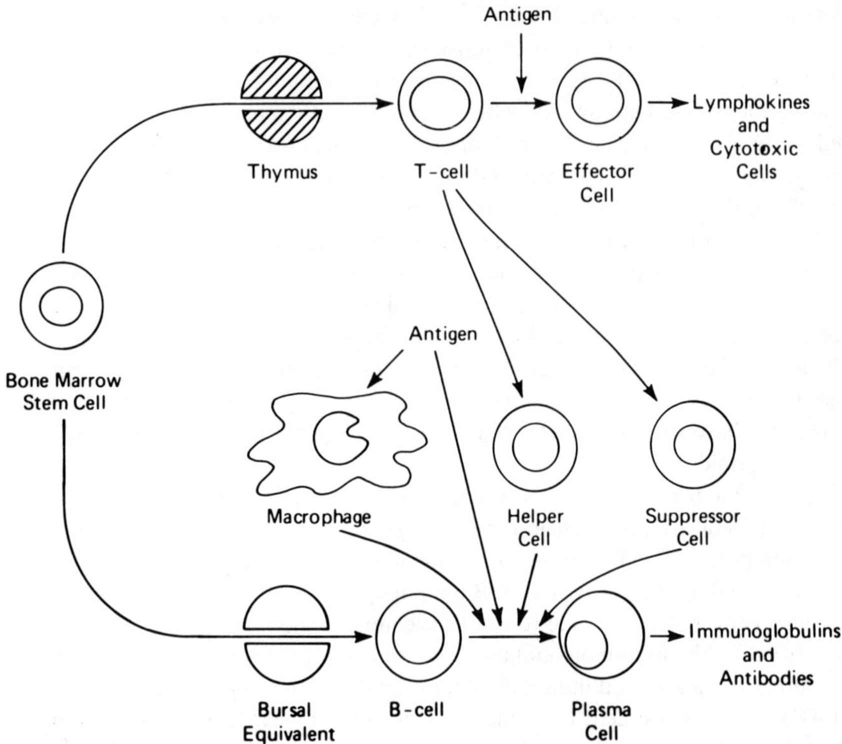

Fig. 1. The two-component concept of the development of immunocompetence. Stem cells from the bone marrow that differentiate under the influence of the bursal equivalent become B cells that respond to antigens by synthesizing and secreting antibodies. Those stem cells that receive differentiative influences from the thymus become T cells that respond to antigens by producing lymphokines and cytotoxic lymphocytes. Thymus-derived lymphocytes also exert "helper" and "suppressor" activities on B cells and modulate antibody synthesis.

stage of B-cell maturation, formation of T cells occurs during embryonic life[45] and apparently does not require stimulation by antigen. The role of the thymus in this event has been shown by the development of T cells from bone marrow cells treated with thymus extracts in vitro [46,47] and the appearance of rosette-forming cells in a patient with cellular immune deficiency after thymus transplantation.[48] Presumably, exposure to antigen triggers a second stage of differentiation in which a specific subpopulation of T cells matures to effector cells that synthesize and secrete lymphokines and have direct cytotoxic activities.

Certain of the congenital immunodeficiency syndromes are apparently due to developmental lesions at specific sites in these differentiative pathways (Table 1).

TABLE 1. Lymphocyte Defects in Patients with Selected Immunodeficiency Syndromes

| | Affected Lymphocyte Populations | | | | |
| | T cells | | B cells | | Mode of |
Disorder	Stage 1*	Stage 2*	Stage 1*	Stage 2*	Inheritance
SCID (thymic alymphoplasia)	yes	yes	(yes)†	(yes)	X-linked
SCID (Swiss-type)	yes	yes	(yes)	(yes)	autosomal rescessive
SCID with ADA deficiency	yes	yes	(yes)	(yes)	autosomal recessive
SCID with ectodermal dysplasia and dwarfism	yes	yes	yes	yes	? autosomal recessive
SCID (sporadic)	yes	yes	yes	yes	unknown
Bruton-type hypo-gammaglobulinemia	no	no	yes	yes	X-linked
X-linked immuno-deficiency with nor-mal or hyperglobu-linemia	no	no	(no)	(yes)	X-linked
Common variable hypogamma-globulinemia	no	no	no	yes§	? autosomal recessive
Hypogammaglobu-linemia with thymoma	no	no	no	yes§	unknown
Immunodeficiency with elevated IgM	no	no	no	(yes)	X-linked
IgA deficiency	no	(no)	no	no	variable
Thymus hypoplasia	yes	yes	no	no	unknown
DiGeorge syndrome	yes	yes	no	no	unknown
Chronic mucocutan-eous candidiasis	no	yes	no	no	? autosomal recessive
Ataxia-telangiectasia	(yes)	yes	no	(no)	autosomal recessive
Wiskott-Aldrich syndrome	yes	yes	no	(yes)	X-linked

*Indicates first and second stages of lymphoid cell differentiation (see text).
†Statements enclosed in parentheses indicate defects that are variable in severity or expression.
§Recent evidence indicates a role for suppressor T cells (see text).

Although various syndromes may affect specific cell populations in most patients, these disorders are heterogeneous and there are exceptions to the generalizations in the Table. Furthermore, as new techniques are applied the cellular definitions will almost certainly require revision.

The severe form of combined immunodeficiency (SCID) is apparently due to a defect in production of lymphoid stem cells. There are several forms of this disease including an X-linked recessive form, an autosomal recessive form, an autosomal recessive form associated with deficiency of the enzyme adenosine deaminase (ADA),[49] a form associated with short-limbed dwarfism and ectodermal dysplasia, and a "sporadic" form. It has not been shown that these subtypes have different underlying developmental defects, although such could be inferred by their distinct genetic transmission. Patients with SCID are virtually devoid of both cellular and humoral immune responses and usually have hypogammaglobulinemia and severe lymphopenia affecting both B and T cells, although exceptional patients may have serum immunoglobulins, usually IgM. Patients with SCID are extremely susceptible to infections with common pathogens as well as opportunistic organisms, and death in early life is common.

Several patients with SCID have been restored to immunologic competence by transplantation of genetically-matched bone marrow,[50, 51] and in one case by an infusion of fetal liver cells.[40] If one assumes that these results were due to replacement of the deficient stem cells, then the organs required for differentiation of immunocompetent cells (thymus and bursal equivalent) from stem cells must be functional.

DEFECTS INVOLVING THE B-CELL SYSTEM

Patients with the Bruton-type of X-linked hypogammaglobulinemia have normal cell-mediated immune responses, but antibody and immunoglobulin synthesis are deficient. These patients usually lack B cells.[40] According to the model in Figure 1, patients with this disease possess stem cells, but apparently lack the "bursal equivalent" necessary for differentiation of stem cells into B cells.

The common variable form of hypogammaglobulinemia is unique in that the patients are clinically normal during childhood, but develop recurrent infections and evidence of immunodeficiency during adult years. Information from Swedish birth records[52] and studies of lymphocytes from relatives of these patients[53] have suggested that genetic factors may predispose one to development of this disorder. Cellular immune responses in these patients are usually normal.

Of particular interest in this disease is the finding that the patients usually have normal numbers of B lymphocytes. Thus, the antigen-independent first stage of lymphocyte differentiation is apparently intact, but the antigen-dependent second stage is abnormal. A possible explanation for the late onset of this disease is suggested by the recent report by Waldmann et al,[54] who found that when peripheral blood lymphocytes from patients with common variable hypogammaglobulinemia were co-cultured with PWM-stimulated cells from normal donors, secretion of immunoglobulins by the normal cells was markedly suppressed. The cells that possessed the suppressor activity were T cells. After removal of these cells, the B cells from the hypogammaglobulinemia patients were able to secrete immunoglobulins. This suggests that common variable hypogammaglobulinemia may be a disease with defective regulation of T-cell function in which the B cells are affected secondarily. A similar phenomenon of T-cell mediated suppression of immunoglobulin synthesis in vitro has recently been observed in patients with the syndrome of thymoma and hypogammaglobulinemia.[55]

The "dysgammaglobulinemias" are a group of disorders in which the levels of some immunoglobulins are deficient while the concentrations of others are normal or elevated. These patients are usually immunodeficient, and in some cases the immunoglobulins are devoid of antibody activity. In one form, the serum IgM is quite high while IgA and IgG levels are subnormal. One patient with this syndrome had normal numbers of IgM-, IgA- and IgG-bearing B cells suggesting that the defect in this disorder is selective and involves terminal differentiation of some but not all populations of immunoglobulin-secreting cells.[40]

Isolated deficiency of IgA is a commonly recognized laboratory abnormality occurring in about 1 in 500 normal people.[56] In most cases the abnormality occurs sporadically, although there are family studies in which the defect was transmitted as either a dominant or a recessive trait. The patients have normal numbers of IgA-bearing B cells, and when their cells are stimulated with PWM, they synthesize cytoplasmic immunoglobulin in a normal manner.[40] Thus, the synthetic and secretory processes in these cells are intact, but under usual conditions they fail to secrete IgA.

DEFECTS INVOLVING THE T-CELL SYSTEM

Definition of developmental defects of the thymus-dependent system has occurred only recently. The DiGeorge[57] and Nezelof syndromes[58] are due to congenital absence of the thymus, the organ required for maturation of marrow stem cells to T cells. Immunoglobulin and antibody synthesis by these patients are apparently normal but cellular immune responses are deficient. In several patients, thymus transplantation has been followed by the appearance of T cells in the patients' peripheral blood,[48] and in 2 patients this procedure has produced long-lasting restoration of immunocompetence.[59,60] One patient with isolated T-cell deficiency has been shown to have a deficiency of the enzyme purine nucleoside phosphorylase.[61] This finding is of interest because this enzyme is in the same metabolic pathway as ADA.

In other patients, the number of T cells is normal and the functional defect involves maturation of effector cells in response to antigenic stimulation. These patients are often infected with Candida albicans in a unique syndrome that only involves the skin, nails, and mucous membranes and which is resistant to chemotherapy.[62] Delayed skin responses to candida and other naturally encountered antigens are usually absent. In addition, blood lymphocytes from many of the patients do not respond to in vitro stimulation with antigens, especially candida, by producing lymphokines or by replication. In some respects these patients are functionally analogous to patients with the common variable type of hypogammaglobulinemia; they have achieved the first stage of T-cell differentiation, but are unable to respond in the antigen-dependent stage. The possible role of suppressor cells in these patients is currently under investigation.

Other immunodeficiency syndromes are more complex and have defects involving both B- and T-cell lines. Patients with ataxia-telangiectasia are usually anergic and have deficient numbers of T cells.[40,63] Moreover, they often have severe IgA deficiency even though they have normal numbers of IgA-bearing B cells that secrete immunoglobulin into the cytoplasm when stimulated with PWM. Certain immunologic features of this syndrome are similar to congenitally athymic "nude" mice which also lack T cells and serum IgA, but have normal numbers of IgA-bearing B cells.

The Wiskott-Aldrich syndrome is an X-linked disorder with severe immunodeficiency, thrombocytopenia and eczema.[64,65] Deficient T-cell functions and lymphopenia are common and serum immunoglobulins, especially IgE and IgM, are usually abnormal. A unique feature of this disorder is the marked impairment of antibody responses to polysaccharide antigens.

CANCER IN PATIENTS WITH PRIMARY IMMUNODEFICIENCY SYNDROMES

Coincident with the developing knowledge of the pathogenesis of immunodeficiency syndromes were case reports in which malignant diseases also occurred in patients with primary immune deficiencies.[66] In the early 1970s, the reports from laboratories with large numbers of immunodeficient patients clearly demonstrated an increased incidence of malignant tumors in these subjects and showed that leukemias and lymphoreticular neoplasms were most frequently encountered.[67,68] Gatti and Good[67] estimated that the incidence of malignancy in patients with primary immunodeficiencies may be 10,000 times higher than a comparable control population. Recently, Kersey et al[69] collected 60 instances of fatal cancer in immunodeficient patients under 15 years of age. The total number of immunodeficient patients seen by the contributing physicians was approximately 700, and the mortality rate was 0.8 deaths per 100 patients per year. According to Miller,[70] the mortality for cancer in children of the same age group is 0.007 deaths per 100 patients per year. Thus, the risk in the immunodeficient subjects was 100 times that of the controls.

Recently, a Registry was established to facilitate collection of information on the histologic type and location of cancers in immunodeficient patients. The results of the study were tabulated in 1973[71] and these data are summarized in Table 2. Of the 151 tumors reported to the Registry, 88 (58%) involved the tumors of lymphoreticular system. These neoplasms accounted for the majority of cancers in patients with isolated IgM deficiency (83%), the Wiskott-Aldrich syndrome (79%), ataxia-telangiectasia (62%), common variable hypogammaglobulinemia (56%) and SCID (67%). An estimate of the frequency of tumors in the various patient populations is shown in Table 3. With the exception of SCID in which the risk was approximately 2%, the risk in other disorders was extremely high, ranging from 6 to 10%. These figures are even more striking when one considers the fact that these patients often have shorter life spans because of intercurrent infections.

A recent report from the Registry (kindly provided by Ms. Beatrice Spector) showed that the frequency distributions for most of the immunodeficiencies was unchanged. The notable exception was X-linked hypogammaglobulinemia in which lymphoreticular tumors occurred in 6 patients (43%), leukemia in 7 (50%) and a central nervous system tumor was reported once.

Additional evidence for a relationship between immunodeficiencies and cancer has come from examination of mortality figures (Table 4). Lymphomas were responsible for 69% of the cancer deaths in immunodeficient patients, but only 8% in a control group.[69]

The data in Table 2 also show that certain malignancies occur more frequently in association with certain immunodeficiencies. Five of the disorders in which the serum IgM levels were abnormal (SCID, IgM deficiency, X-linked hypogammaglobulinemia, common variable hypogammaglobulinemia, and the Wiskott-Aldrich syndrome) were associated with lymphoreticular neoplasms (59 tumors in 94 patients). In constrast, epithelial tumors were the most frequently observed types in patients with isolated IgA deficiency and in 5 of 9 cases the tumors arose in the epithelium of the gut. Of the 32 lymphoreticular neoplasms in patients with ataxia-telangiectasia, 11 were lymphosarcomas, 7 were reticulum cell sarcomas, and 7 were malignant lymphomas. Patients with the Wiskott-Aldrich syndrome develop a poorly differentiated reticuloendotheliosis (8 cases among 19 lymphoreticular tumors) and this tumor often involves the brain.

It is well-established that neonatal thymectomy markedly enhances the susceptibility of animals to viral- and chemical-induced neoplasia.[72] There is also general agreement that cell-mediated immune responses provide the major immunologic mechanism for destruction of foreign tissues, including tumors.[73] It is, therefore, of considerable interest that the Registry has recorded no instances of cancer in patients with immunologic defects that were limited to the T-cell system. Whether this is due to the relative difficulty of diagnosis of

TABLE 2. Malignancies in Patients With Primary Immunodeficiency Diseases*

Disease	Epithelial No.	(%)	Lympho-reticular No.	(%)	Leukemia No.	(%)	Mesen-chymal No.	(%)	Nervous System No.	(%)	Total tumors
SCID	0		6	(67)	3	(33)	0		0		9
X-linked hypogamma-globulinemia	0		1	(17)	5	(83)	0		0		6
IgM deficiency	0		5	(83)	0		0		1	(17)	6
IgA deficiency	9	(69)	2	(15)	0		1	(8)	1	(8)	13
Common variable immunodeficiency	12	(29)	23	(56)	4	(10)	1	(2)	1	(2)	41
Wiskott-Aldrich syndrome	0		19	(79)	3	(13)	1	(4)	1	(4)	24
Ataxia-telangiectasia	6	(11)	32	(62)	11	(21)	1	(2)	2	(4)	52

*Data on Tables 2 and 3 from Kersey, J. H., Spector, B. D. and Good, R. A.: Primary immunodeficiency diseases and cancer: The Immunodeficiency Cancer Registry. Int. J. Cancer 12:333, 1973, with permission.

TABLE 3. Incidence of Malignancy in Primary Immunodeficiency Syndromes*

Disease	Approximate Incidence	Approximate Risk
SCID	9/approx 400	2%
X-linked hypogamma-globulinemia	6/approx 100	6%
IgM deficiency	6/approx 70	8%
Common variable hypogammaglobulinemia	41/approx 500	8%
Wiskott-Aldrich syndrome	24/approx 300	8%
Ataxia-telangiectasia	52/approx 500	10%

*Data from Kersey et al [71]

TABLE 4. Cancers in Control Subjects and Patients with Primary Immunodeficiencies*

Tumor	Control† %	Immunodeficient %
Leukemias (all types)	48	25
Central nervous system	16	3
Lymphomas (all types)	8	69
Bone	4	0
Other	24	3

*Data from Kersey, J. H., Spector, B. D. and Good, R. A.: Cancer in children with primary immunodeficiency diseases. J. Pediatr. 84:263, 1974, with permission.
†Data from Miller, R. W.: Fifty-two forms of childhood cancer: United States mortality experience, 1960–1966. J. Pediatr. 75:685, 1969, with permission.

diseases affecting T-cell function or to early deaths of these patients from infections or other complications rather than cancer is unknown.

Although mucocutaneous candidiasis is a heterogeneous disorder and occurs in a variety of immunodeficient settings, it is often a hallmark of defective cell-mediated immunity. It has occurred in patients with the DiGeorge,[57,59,60] and Nezelof[48] syndromes which represent extreme forms of T-cell immunodeficiency. However, patients with the more common forms of mucocutaneous candidiasis have normal numbers of T cells (C. H. Kirkpatrick, unpublished), but their lymphocytes are unable to develop normal cell-mediated immune responses to candida antigens.[62] Indeed, 20 of the 28 candidiasis patients studied at the NIH had cellular immune defects. Yet none of the patients have developed tumors of the histologic types that are common in patients with other immunodeficiency diseases. Instead, there may be a predisposition to development of thymomas. This tumor has occurred in 4 (14%) of our 28 patients, but was recorded only twice (1%) among the 145 immunodeficient patients reported to the Registry.[71] In their recent literature review, Windhorst and Stoltzman[74] found 10 cases of candidiasis with thymomas and, of the 7 patients in whom cellular immunologic studies were done, defects were found in 5.

There may be an analogy between the development of thymoma in patients with this form of cellular immunodeficiency and the occurrence of nodular lymphoid hyperplasia in the intestinal mucosa in patients with common variable hypogammaglobulinemia.[75, 76] In both disorders the first stage of lymphoid cell differentiation is achieved but subsequent antigen-dependent maturation of effector cells is impaired. It is possible that the excessive proliferation of lymphoid cells in these disorders is either a compensatory mechanism, or due to failure of a feedback signal from terminally differentiated cells.

CANCER IN PATIENTS WITH SECONDARY IMMUNODEFICIENCY SYNDROMES

The occurrence of cancer in recipients of immunosuppressive or cytotoxic drugs has recently been reviewed by Penn, who recorded primary tumors in 182 recipients of kidney (180 patients) or cardiac (2 patients) allografts.[77] Epithelial tumors occurred in 129 (67%) patients and the most frequently involved tissues were the skin (57 cases), lip (16 cases), and uterine cervix (15 cases). Sixty patients (33%) had tumors of mesenchymal organs; 53 of these tumors were lymphomas and included 38 reticulum sarcomas.

The overall risk of development of a primary malignancy among the kidney transplant recipients at the University of Colorado Medical Center was 5–6%, approximately 100 times that expected in an age-matched control population.[77]

The frequency and type of neoplasms occurring in renal transplant recipients throughout the world has been reported by Hoover and Fraumeni.[78] In 6297 patients transplanted from 1951–1971 inclusive, the risk of lymphoma was 2.2/1000/year, or 30–40 times the expected value. The risk for reticulum cell sarcoma in the recipients was 350 times that expected in the control group. Of additional interest was the finding that 13 of 25 lymphomas (52%) were localized to the brain; an event that occurred in only 1% of the controls.

Skin cancer was 4 times as frequent in the transplant recipients, but Hoover and Fraumeni point out that many of these cancers occurred in high-risk geographic areas.[78]

Penn also described 47 instances in which organs had been transplanted from cancer-bearing donors into apparently cancer-free recipients.[77] In 10 recipients, the transplanted tumor spread to distant sites and was probably the cause of death in 7 cases. In the remaining patients, the immunosuppressive therapy was stopped and the tumors disappeared, presumably through rejection reactions.

Other evidence suggests that chronic immunosuppressive therapy for chronic inflammatory diseases may also be associated with an increased incidence of malignancy. This is especially noteworthy in psoriasis patients in whom 22 instances of cancer have been recorded. However, in other disorders, particularly autoimmune diseases, it is less certain if neoplasms are complications of the basic diseases or of the immunosuppressive therapy.

DISCUSSION

The evidence reviewed in this paper makes it clear that cancer occurs much more frequently in patients with immunodeficiency diseases than in matched, but immunologically normal, control subjects. These findings could be coincidental and due to an intrinsic predisposition of the patients' tissues to neoplastic transformation in a manner analogous to tissues from patients with Fanconi anemia or Down syndrome.[79, 80] However, when cells from patients with a variety of primary immunodeficiencies were analyzed for susceptibility to transformation by the SV40 virus, no abnormalities were found.[68,81] This suggested that the susceptibility to malignancy was on a different basis and presumably involved the immunologic functions that inactivate potentially oncogenic agents or toxins or destroy transformed cells.

It is of interest that there is no constellation of immunologic defects that clearly predisposes patients to neoplasia. Neoplasms occur in patients with "dysgammaglobulinemias", pan-hypogammaglobulinemia with normal T-cell functions and mixed immunodeficiencies. Curiously, the Registry has received no reports of cancers in patients with isolated defects in T-cell function. This situation is analogous to "nude" mice with congenital aplasia of the thymus. These mice fail to reject allogenic or xenogenic skin grafts and have supported growth of transplanted human tumors.[82 – 84] Yet spontaneous primary tumors in "nude" mice are extremely rare.[85]

Moreover, these observations indicate the complexity of the defense mechanisms against cancer. If susceptibility to cancer were simply a problem of defective detection and destruction of tumor cells, one would expect to find an increase in the incidence of all forms of cancer, especially the common childhood tumors such as retinoblastoma, Wilms tumor and neuroblastoma. However, there is no increase in the incidence of these tumors in immunodeficient patients. Instead, most of the tumors in these patients involve the lymphoreticular and hematopoietic systems. Thus, although cellular immune responses with production of lymphokines and cytotoxic lymphocytes are important for destruction of foreign cells, the total surveillance system probably also requires contributions from other systems such as complement and macrophages. In this regard, Snyderman et al have recently reported that loss of monocyte responses to chemotactic stimuli is an early and common defect in cancer-bearing patients and animals.[86]

It is well known that many experimental tumors are caused by viruses[3,4,7] and Schwartz[87] has proposed a mechanism through which defects in immunologic responses may predispose one to virus-mediated tumors.[87] He has suggested that immunodeficient patients lack the "feedback loops" that control immune responses such as lymphocyte transformation and that sustained proliferation of lymphoid cells in response to new tissue antigens results in lymphoid tumors. This mechanism would explain the frequency of lymphoreticular neoplasms in immunodeficient patients. Presumably, a similar phenomenon could account for tumors that are induced by other carcinogens.

ACKNOWLEDGMENT

The author is indebted to Ms. Beatrice Spector of the Immunodeficiency-Cancer Registry for providing current data. Persons interested in contributing to the Registry should contact Ms. Spector or Dr. John H. Kersey, Dept. of Lab Medicine and Pathology, Box 609, Mayo Memorial Bldg., Minneapolis, MN 55455.

REFERENCES

1. Thomas, L.: Open discussion. In Lawrence, H. S. (Ed.): "Cellular and Humoral Aspects of Hypersensitivity States." New York: H. Hoeber, 1959, pp. 529–532.
2. Burnet, F. M.: "Immunological Surveillance." Oxford: Pergamon Press, 1970.
3. Allen, D. W. and Cole, P.: Viruses and human cancer. N. Engl. J. Med. 286:70, 1972.
4. Sjögren, H. O. and Bansal, S. C.: Antigens in virally induced tumors. In Amos, B. (Ed.): "Progress in Immunology." New York: Academic Press, Inc., 1971, pp. 921–938.
5. Prehn, R. T. and Main, J. M.: Immunity to methylcholanthrene-induced sarcomas. J. Natl. Cancer Inst. 18:769, 1957.
6. Klein, G.: Tumor-specific transplantation antigens. Cancer Res. 28:625, 1968.
7. Smith, R. T.: Tumor-specific immune mechanisms. N. Engl. J. Med. 278:1207, 1268 and 1326, 1968.
8. Ryser, H. J.-P.: Chemical carcinogenesis. N. Engl. J. Med. 285:721, 1971.
9. Halterman, R. H., Leventhal, B. G. and Mann, D. L.: An acute-leukemia antigen: Correlation with clinical status. N. Engl. J. Med. 287:1272, 1972.
10. Morton, D. A. and Malmgren, R. A.: Human osteosarcomas. Immunologic evidence suggesting an associated infectious agent. Science 162:1279, 1968.
11. Byers, V. S., Levin, A. S., Hackett, A. J. and Fudenberg, H. H.: Tumor-specific cell-mediated immunity in household contacts of cancer patients. J. Clin. Invest. 55: 500, 1975.
12. Morton, D. L., Malmgren, R. A. and Holmes, E. C.: Demonstration of antibodies against human malignant melanoma by immunofluorescence. Surgery 64:233, 1968.
13. Hellstrom, I. and Hellstrom, K. E.: Some recent studies on cellular immunity to melanomas. Fed. Proc. 32:156, 1973.
14. Char, D. H., Hollinshead, A., Cogan, D. G. et al: Cutaneous delayed hypersensitivity reactions to soluble melanoma antigen in patients with ocular malignant melanoma. N. Engl. J. Med. 291:274, 1974.
15. Fass, L., Herberman, R. B. and Ziegler, J.: Delayed cutaneous hypersensitivity to autologous extracts of Burkitt-lymphoma cells. N. Engl. J. Med. 282:776, 1970.

16. Abelev, G. L.: Alpha-fetoprotein in ontogenesis and its association with malignant tumors. Adv. Cancer Res. 14:295, 1971.
17. Hellstrom, I., Hellstrom, K. E., Pierce, G. E. and Bill, A. H.: Demonstration of cell-bound and humoral immunity against neuroblastoma cells. Proc. Natl. Acad. Sci. USA 60:1231, 1968.
18. Gold, P. and Freedman, S. O.: Specific carcinoembryonic antigens of the human digestive system. J. Exp. Med. 122:467, 1965.
19. Herberman, R. B.: In vivo and in vitro assays of cellular immunity to tumor antigens. Fed. Proc. 32:160, 1973.
20. Jehn, V. W., Nathanson, L., Schwartz, R. S. and Skinner, M.: In vitro lymphocyte stimulation by a soluble antigen from malignant melanoma. N. Engl. J. Med. 283: 329, 1970.
21. Fefer, A., Mickelson, E. and Thomas, E. D.: Leukemia antigens: Mixed leukocyte culture tests on twelve leukemic patients with identical twins. Clin. Exp. Immunol. 18: 237, 1974.
22. Mavligit, G. M., Hersh, E. M. and McBride, C. M.: Lymphocyte blastogenesis induced by autochthonous human solid tumor cells: Relationship to stage of disease and serum factors. Cancer 34:1712, 1974.
23. Bloom, B., Bennett, B., Oettgen, H. F. et al: Demonstration of delayed hypersensitivity to soluble antigens of chemically induced tumors by inhibition of macrophage migration. Proc. Natl. Acad. Sci. USA 64:1176, 1969.
24. Churchill, W. H., Zbar, B., Belli, J. A. and David, J. R.: Detection of cellular immunity to tumor antigens of a guinea pig hepatoma by inhibition of macrophage migration. J. Natl. Cancer Inst. 48:541, 1972.
25. Hilberg, R. W., Balcerzak, S. P. and LoBuglio, A. F.: A migration inhibition-factor assay for tumor immunity in man. Cell. Immunol. 7:152, 1973.
26. McIllmurray, M. B., Price, M. R. and Langman, M. J. S.: Inhibition of leukocyte migration in patients with large intestinal cancer by extracts prepared from large intestinal tumors and from normal colonic mucosa. Br. J. Cancer 29:305, 1974.
27. Perlman, P., O'Toole, C. and Unsgaard, B.: Cell-mediated immune mechanisms of tumor cell destruction. Fed. Proc. 32:153, 1973.
28. Bennett, B.: Specific suppression of tumor growth by isolated peritoneal macrophages from immunized mice. J. Immunol. 95:656, 1965.
29. Jurin, M. and Suit, H. D.: Transfer of resistence to tumor with lymphoid cells from immunized allogeneic donors. Tex. Rep. Biol. Med. 31:29, 1973.
30. Nadler, S. H. and Moore, G. E.: Immunotherapy of malignant disease. Arch. Surg. 99:376, 1969.
31. Klein, E., Holtermann, O. A., Case, R. W. et al: Responses of neoplasms to local immunotherapy, Am. J. Clin. Pathol. 62:281, 1974.
32. Bast, R. C., Zbar, B., Borsos, T. and Rapp, H. J.: BCG and cancer. N. Engl. J. Med. 290: 1413 and 1458, 1974.
33. Sokal, J. E., Aungst, C. W. and Snyderman, M.: Delay in progression of malignant lymphoma after BCG vaccination. N. Engl. J. Med. 291:1226, 1974.
34. Hellstrom, I., Hellstrom, K. E., Evans, C. A. et al: Serum-mediated protection of neoplastic cells from inhibition by lymphocytes immune to their tumor-specific antigens. Proc. Natl. Acad. Sci. USA 62:362, 1969.
35. Stutman, O.: Carcinogen-induced immune depression: Absence in mice resistant to chemical oncogenesis. Science 166:620, 1969.
36. Friedman, H. and Ceglowski, W. S.: Cellular basis for the immunosuppressive properties of a leukaemogenic virus. Nature 218:1232, 1968.

37. Bruton, O. C.: Agammaglobulinemia. Pediatrics 9:722, 1952.
38. Cooper, M. D., Perey, D. Y., Peterson, R. D. A. et al: The two-component concept of the lymphoid system. In Bergsma, D. (Ed.): "Immunologic Deficiency Diseases in Man," Birth Defects: Orig. Art. Ser., vol. IV, no. 1. White Plains: The National Foundation—March of Dimes, 1968, p. 7.
39. Cooper, M. D. and Lawton, A. R.: Circulating B cells in patients with immuno-deficiency. Am. J. Pathol. 69:513, 1972.
40. Cooper, M. D., Keightley, R. G., Wu, L. Y. F. and Lawton, A. R.: Development defects of T and B cell lines in humans. Transplant. Rev. 16:51, 1973.
41. Jondal, M., Wigzell, H. and Aiuti, F.: Human lymphocyte subpopulations: Classification according to surface markers and/or functional characteristics. Transplant. Rev. 16:163, 1973.
42. Katz, D. H. and Benacerraf, B.: The regulatory influence of activated T cells on B cell responses to antigen. Adv. Immunol. 15:1, 1972.
43. Rosenthal, A. S., Blake, J. T., Ellner, J. J. et al: The role of macrophages in T lymphocyte antigen recognition. In Rosenthal, A. S. (Ed.): "Immune Recognition." New York: Academic Press, 1975, pp. 539—554.
44. Wu, L. Y. F., Lawton, A. R. and Cooper, M. D.: Differentiation capacity of cultured B lymphocytes from immunodeficient patients. J. Clin. Invest. 52:3180, 1973.
45. Wybran, J., Carr, M. C. and Fudenberg, H. H.: The human rosette-forming cell as a marker of a population of thymus-derived cells. J. Clin. Invest. 51:2537, 1972.
46. Komuro, K. and Boyse, E. A.: In-vitro demonstration of thymic hormone in the mouse by conversion of precursor cells into lymphocytes. Lancet 1:740, 1973.
47. Incefy, G. S., L'Esperance, P. and Good, R. A.: In vitro differentiation of human marrow cells into T lymphocytes by thymic extracts using the rosette technique. Clin. Exp. Immunol. 19:475, 1975.
48. Kirkpatrick, C. H., Ottesen, E. A., Smith, T. K. et al: Reconstitution of defective cellular immunity with fetal thymus and dialyzable transfer factor: Long term studies in a patient with chronic mucocutaneous candidiasis. Clin. Exp. Immunol. (In press).
49. Parkman, R., Gelfand, E. W., Rosen, F. S. et al: Severe combined immunodeficiency and adenosine deaminase deficiency. N. Engl. J. Med. 292:714, 1975.
50. Van Bekkum, D. W.: Use and abuse of hemopoietic cell grafts in immune deficiency diseases. Transplant. Rev. 9:3, 1972.
51. Good, R. A.: Highlights of the workshop on primary immunodeficiencies: Where have we been — where are we going? In Bergsma, D. (Ed.): "Immunodeficiency in Man and Animals," Birth Defects: Orig. Art. Ser., vol. XI, no. 1. Sunderland, MA: Sinauer Associates, Inc., for The National Foundation—March of Dimes, 1975, pp. 579—591.
52. Wollheim, F. A., Belfrage, S., Coster, C. and Lindholm, H.: Primary "acquired" hypo-gammaglobulinemia. Acta Med. Scand. 176:1, 1964.
53. Kamin, R. M., Fudenberg, H. H. and Douglas, S. D.: A genetic defect in "acquired" agammaglobulinemia. Proc. Natl. Acad. Sci. USA 60:881, 1968.
54. Waldmann, T. A., Durm, M., Broder, S. et al: Role of suppressor T cells in pathogenesis of common variable hypogammaglobulinemia. Lancet 2:609, 1974.
55. Waldmann, T. A. Broder, S., Durm, M. et al: The role of suppressor T cells in the pathogenesis of hypogammaglobulinemia with a thymoma. Clin. Res. 23:447A, 1975.
56. Collins-Williams, C., Kokubu, H. L., Lamenza, C. et al: Incidence of isolated deficiency of IgA in the serum of Canadian children. Ann. Allergy 30:11, 1972.
57. DiGeorge, A. M.: Congenital absence of the thymus and its immunologic consequences: Concurrence with congenital hypoparathyroidism. In "Immunologic Deficiency Diseases in Man," op. cit., pp. 116—123.

58. Nezelof, C.: Thymic dysplasia with normal immunoglobulins and immunologic deficiency: Pure alymphocytosis, ibid, pp. 104–112.
59. August, C. S., Levey, R. H., Berkel, A. J. and Rosen, F. S.: Establishment of immunological competence in a child with congenital thymic aplasia by a graft of fetal thymus. Lancet 1:1080, 1970.
60. Cleveland, W. W.: Immunologic reconstitution in the DiGeorge syndrome by fetal thymic transplant. In "Immunodeficiency in Man and Animals," op. cit., pp. 352–356.
61. Giblett, E. R., Ammann, A. J., Wara, D. W. et al: Nucleoside-phosphorylase deficiency in a child with severely defective T-cell immunity and normal B-cell immunity. Lancet 1:1010, 1975.
62. Kirkpatrick, C. H., Rich, R. R. and Bennett, J. E.: Chronic mucocutaneous candidiasis: Model-building in cellular immunity. Ann. Intern. Med. 74:955, 1971.
63. Biggar, W. D. and Good, R. A.: Immunodeficiency in ataxia-telangiectasia. In "Immunodeficiency in Man and Animals," op. cit., pp. 271–276.
64. Blaese, R. M., Strober, W., Brown, R. S. and Waldmann, T. A.: The Wiskott-Aldrich syndrome. A disorder with a possible defect in antigen processing or recognition. Lancet 1:1056, 1968.
65. Cooper, M. D., Chase, H. P., Lowman, J. T. et al: Wiskott-Aldrich syndrome. An immunologic deficiency disease involving the afferent limb of immunity. Am. J. Med. 44:499, 1968.
66. Page, A. R., Hansen, A. E. and Good, R. A.: Occurrence of leukemia and lymphoma in patients with agammaglobulinemia. Blood 21:197, 1963.
67. Gatti, R. A. and Good, R. A.: Occurrence of malignancy in immunodeficiency diseases. Cancer 28:89, 1971.
68. Waldman, T. A., Strober, W. and Blaese, R. M.: Immunodeficiency disease and malignancy. Ann. Intern. Med. 77:605, 1972.
69. Kersey, J. H., Spector, B. D., and Good, R. A.: Cancer in children with primary immunodeficiency diseases. J. Pediatr. 84:263, 1974.
70. Miller, R. W.: Fifty-two forms of childhood cancer: United States mortality experience, 1960–1966. J. Pediatr. 75:685, 1969.
71. Kersey, J. H., Spector, B. D. and Good, R.A.: Primary immunodeficiency diseases and cancer: The Immunodeficiency Cancer Registry. Int. J. Cancer 12:333, 1973.
72. Kersey, J. H., Spector, B. D. and Good, R. A.: Immunodeficiency and cancer. Adv. Cancer Res. 18:211, 1973.
73. Good, R. A.: Relations between immunity and malignancy. Proc. Natl. Acad. Sci. USA 69:1026, 1972.
74. Windhorst, D. and Stoltzner, G.: Candidiasis in thymoma. In "Proc. Third International Conference on Mycoses." Washington, D.C.: Pan American Health Org. Sci. Pub., 304. (In press).
75. Hermans, P. E., Huizenga, K. A., Hoffman, H. N. et al: Dysgammaglobulinemina associated with nodular lymphoid hyperplasia of the small intestine. Am. J. Med. 40:78, 1966.
76. Kirkpatrick, C. H., Waxman, D., Smith, O. D. and Schimke, R. N.: Hypogammaglobulinemia with nodular lymphoid hyperplasia of the small bowel. Arch. Intern. Med. 121: 273, 1968.
77. Penn, I.: Occurrence of cancer in immunodeficiencies. Cancer (Suppl.) 34:858, 1974.
78. Hoover, R. and Fraumeni, J. F.: Risk of cancer in renal-transplant recipients. Lancet 2:55, 1973.
79. Todaro, G. J., Green, H. and Swift, M. R.: Susceptibility of human diploid fibroblast strains to transformation by SV40 virus. Science 153:1252, 1966.

80. Todaro, G. J. and Martin, G.: Increased susceptibility of Down's syndrome fibroblasts to transformation by SV40. Proc. Soc. Exp. Biol. Med. 124:1232, 1967.

81. Kersey, J. H., Gatti, R. A., Good, R. A. et al: Susceptibility of cells from patients with primary immunodeficiency to transformation with Simian virus 40. Proc. Natl. Acad. Sci. USA 69:980, 1972.

82. Pantelouris, E. M.: Observations on the immunobiology of "nude" mice. Immunology 20:247, 1971.

83. Poulsen, C. O. and Rygaard, J.: Heterotransplantation of human adenocarcinomas of the colon and rectum to the mouse mutant nude. A study of nine consecutive transplantations. Acta Pathol. Microbiol. Scand. (A) 79:159, 1971.

84. Rygaard, J. and Poulsen, C. O.: Heterotransplantation of a human tumor to "nude" mice. Acta Pathol. Microbiol. Scand. 77:758, 1969.

85. Custer, R. P., Outzen, H. C., Eaton, G. J. and Prehn, R. T.: Does the absence of immunologic surveillance affect the tumor incidence in "nude" mice? First recorded spontaneous lymphoma in a "nude" mouse. J. Natl. Cancer Inst. 51:707, 1973.

86. Snyderman, R., Pike, M. C., Meadows, L. et al: Depression of monocyte chemotaxis by neoplasms. Clin. Res. 23:297A, 1975.

87. Schwartz, R. S.: Immunoregulation, oncogenic viruses and malignant lymphomas. Lancet 1:1266, 1972.

Delayed Mutation as a Cause of Retinoblastoma: Application to Genetic Counseling[*]

Jürgen Herrmann, MD

INTRODUCTION

Delayed mutation has been considered a possible cause of ectrodactyly,[1] achondroplasia,[2,3] the Wiedemann-Beckwith syndrome[3,4] and retinoblastoma.[5] The concept of delayed mutation was developed by Charlotte Auerbach on the basis of chemically induced mutations in Drosophila[6] and was then used by her to explain the sudden occurrence of the same autosomal dominant mutation (ectrodactyly) in several distantly related members of one family.[1] The clinical, developmental and genetic implications of this concept were recently pointed out by Herrmann and Opitz.[3]

The model of delayed mutation involves 2 consecutive mutational processes at a single locus with an unstable "premutated" allele which is distinct from and intermediate to the normal (wild) and the (fully) mutated allele. We have called the change from the wild to the premutated allele *premutation* and the change from the premutated to the mutated allele we have termed *telomutation*. The phenotype associated with the premutated allele may or may not be abnormal; in man it has been normal for all conditions investigated so far.

The model is particularly well suited to explain the sudden occurrence of the same autosomal dominant condition in several branches of one family, but the model also allows for occurrence of an autosomal dominant condition in not-so-distant relatives, such as in sibs with unaffected parents, in an uncle and his niece etc. The model does not preclude the occurrence of sporadic cases which, in fact, may be frequent, especially in traits with low fitness. Delayed mutation, therefore, may be suspected when a condition shows dominant transmission in

*Supported by USPHS/NIH grant GM 20130. Paper no. 1888 from the University of Wisconsin Genetics Laboratory.

Birth Defects: Original Article Series, Volume XII, Number 1, pages 79–90

some families, occurs in a single sibship in other families, is observed in still other families to affect distantly related individuals, and is also noted in multiple instances to occur as a sporadic case. In this paper we would like to point out some aspects of the model of delayed mutation for counseling situations in retinoblastoma.

SUMMARY OF GENETIC DATA

The genetic data on retinoblastoma have been summarized repeatedly, including recent reviews by Warburg[7] and by François et al.[8] The incidence is most frequently quoted to be slightly less than 1:20,000[7-12] with a range between 1:16,000 and 1:82,000.[13] In Holland,[14] Finland[13] and in Russia[15] a gradual increase in the frequency of retinoblastoma has been documented. Warburg[7] presumes that this increase is mainly due to an increase in bilateral tumors. In Denmark, the incidence of unilateral cases has been estimated as 1:25,000 and the incidence of bilateral cases as 1:61,000.[12]

The mutation rate is estimated to be in the range of $4-6 \times 10^{-6}$ by most authors,[9,11,16] but Schappert-Kimmijser et al[14] calculated a higher rate (1.23×10^{-5}) for the Dutch population. The incidence of the tumor is possibly slightly higher in males than in females.[8,12,14] Initial investigations failed to demonstrate an age effect for retinoblastoma,[17,18] but more recent studies show an increased paternal age particularly for sporadic bilateral cases.[8,11,19] Consanguinity of various degree was seen by Hemmes[20] in 3 of 48 sporadic cases and by Schappert-Kimmijser et al[14] in 9 of 360 sporadic cases. Gordon found a history of consanguinity in 2 of 114 index cases.[21] Reports on the proportion of familial cases were summarized by François et al[8] and found to be 5.13%; most other authors report a familial incidence of roughly 10%.[9,11,14,22] The proportion of familial cases is higher among bilateral than among unilateral cases; in the series of Briard-Guillemot et al[9] the proportions were 17.7% and 6.5%, respectively. Bilateral occurrence is found by most authors in about 30% of sporadic cases and in about 60% of familial cases,[9,11,12,14,23,24] but one report indicates bilateral occurrence in almost 90% of familial cases.[8]

Chromosome studies by the conventional and the newer banding techniques have been informative in several instances. Czeizel et al[25] found multiple nonspecific chromosome aberrations, including aneuploidy, chromatid breaks and chromosome deletions in each of the 12 patients they investigated. A special relationship between the occurrence of retinoblastoma and abnormalities of chromosome 13 has been known for several years[26,27] and has been interpreted to involve an interstitial deletion of the band q21.[28,29] Some, but not all of the patients with this deletion had associated physical abnormalities and mental retardation. Another specific chromosome aberration associated with retinoblastoma is trisomy 21. Of the 5 cases reported in the literature,[30] 2 were doubly aneuploid; one was 48,XXX, 21+, and the other one was 48,XXY,21 +. In addition to those 5 cases, we are personally aware of 2 further cases of the Down syndrome with retinoblastoma. We also know of a case of trisomy 13 with retinoblastoma or a retinoblastoma-like retinal dysplasia.[31]

Another important genetic aspect of retinoblastoma is the increased occurrence of extraocular tumors in retinoblastoma patients and in their close relatives.[5] This association was first pointed out by Jensen and Miller[32] and strongly confirmed subsequently by Kitchin and Ellsworth.[33] The data suggest that in about 1—5% of cases an extraocular tumor may be a pleiotropic manifestation of the retinoblastoma gene; this value may be higher for bilateral and lower for unilateral cases. The method of ascertainment obviously implied that the extraocular tumors occurred later than the retinoblastoma. It was significant, however, that the majority of tumors were osteogenic sarcomas.

OFFSPRING OF AFFECTED INDIVIDUALS

The literature includes compiled data on the offspring of sporadic cases of retinoblastoma and indicates a clear difference for sporadic unilateral affected (SU) vs sporadic bilateral affected (SB) individuals. Vogel compiled a series of 135 SU parents who had a total of 290 normal and 21 affected offspring.[10] An essentially similar and partially overlapping series was produced by François et al.[8] Briard-Guillemot et al[9] found 41 SU parents to have 81 normal and 1 affected offspring. Gordon found 6 SU parents to have 11 normal and 2 affected children.[21] The incidence of affected children is significantly higher among offspring of SB parents. François et al found 28 SB parents to have 23 normal and 25 affected children[8]; Briard-Guillemot et al found 8 SB parents with 4 normal and 5 affected offspring[9]; and Gordon found 5 SB parents with 6 normal and 2 affected offspring. [21]

To obtain comparable figures for offspring of familial cases we recently reviewed all familial instances of retinoblastoma published in the literature.[5] We found 40 families where only sibs were affected (*Group A*), 68 families where consecutive generations were affected (*Group B*), and 27 pedigrees where more distant relatives were affected and the pedigrees indicated transmission through at least 2 unaffected carriers (*Group C*). The pedigrees include at least 85 instances of male-to-male transmission. The affected individuals in the 3 groups showed no significant statistical differences with respect to bilaterally and unilaterally affected males and females, male:female ratio or unilateral:bilateral tumor occurrence. In each group there was a preponderance of males, which, however, was statistically not significant.

The essential data with respect to the offspring of familial unilaterally affected (FU) parents, familial bilaterally affected (FB) parents and of carriers are summarized in Tables 1 and 2. There is a significant difference in the offspring of

TABLE 1. Familial Cases of Retinoblastoma: Offspring of Affected Individuals

Cases	Total	Group B	Group C	M	F	U	B
Parent							
number	77	71	6	46	30	57	18
Offspring							
Normal	104	98	6	73	31	87	17
Male	110	101	9	71	39	81	28
Female	87	82	5	57	30	66	21
Sex unknown	35	35	0	26	7	29	6
Affected	125	120	5	79	44	86	38
Unilateral	36	33	3	21	15	30	5
Bilateral	87	85	2	56	31	55	32
Site unknown	2	2	0	2	0	1	1
Carrier	3	0	3	2	1	3	0

TABLE 2. Familial Cases of Retinoblastoma: Offspring of Unaffected Carriers

Cases	Total	Group A	Group B	Group C	M	F
Parent						
number	138	40	5	93	38	28
Offspring						
Normal	366	93	5	268	117	81
Male	286	73	12	201	83	46
Female	211	61	7	143	63	27
Sex unknown	174	80	0	94	34	45
Affected	244	121	14	109	51	24
Unilateral	86	39	7	40	21	6
Bilateral	104	52	7	45	24	11
Site unknown	54	30	0	24	6	7
Carrier	61	0	0	61	12	13

FU and FB parents ($p < 0.05$), but not between parents of *Group B* vs *Group C* or between male and female parents. The difference between the offspring of FU and FB parents is due to both an increased number of affected offspring and an increased proportion of bilaterally affected persons among the offspring of FB parents.

The pedigrees in *Group A* are selected for an increased number of affected individuals in the sibship and against a high number of carriers. There is, accordingly, a significant difference in the proportion of affected persons among the offspring of carriers in *Group* (s) *A* (and *B*) vs *Group C*. But since the proportion of male:female offspring and unilaterally:bilaterally affected offspring is similar for the carriers in the 3 groups we assume that the carriers constitute a biologically homogeneous class.

In Table 3 the relative proportions of affected and normal offspring of SU, SB, FU, FB, and carrier parents are compared. The offspring of carriers and the offspring of SU parents each appear to form a distinct class. Unfortunately, for SU and SB parents the proportion of unilaterally vs bilaterally affected offspring is not available. It was indicated above that the difference between the offspring of FU parents and the offspring of FB parents is significant.

INTERPRETATION

Interpretation of the genetic data on retinoblastoma according to the model of delayed mutation shows that the mutation at the retinoblastoma locus can occur during mitotic (somatic) or meiotic cell division and that the mutational process can be delayed or complete. For instance, consecutive occurrence in 3 generations of bilaterally affected individuals (Fig. 1, *Pedigree A*) suggests that the mutation was complete-meiotic in the first affected individual and then transmitted according to the rules of autosomal dominant inheritance. An individual case of complete-mitotic mutation is difficult to demonstrate, but the occurrence is supported by the presence of affected individuals who have a large number of unaffected offspring.

TABLE 3. Retinoblastoma: Offspring of Affected and of Carrier Individuals: A Summary

Parent				Offspring		
Type	Affected	U[1]	B[1]	T*	Carrier*	Normal*
SU[2]		–	–	6.8	–	93.2
SB[3]		–	–	52.1	–	47.9
FU		0.35	0.65	49	2	49
FB		0.14	0.86	69	0	31
C		0.45	0.55	36.4	9.1	54.5

Affected parent: SU = Sporadic Unilateral
                   SB = Sporadic Bilateral
                   FU = Familial Unilateral
                   FB = Familial Bilateral
U = unilaterally affected, B = bilaterally affected, T = total number of affected offspring.
*Numbers in %
[1] Relative proportion
[2] Series of Vogel[10] (see text)
[3] Series of François et al[8] (see text)

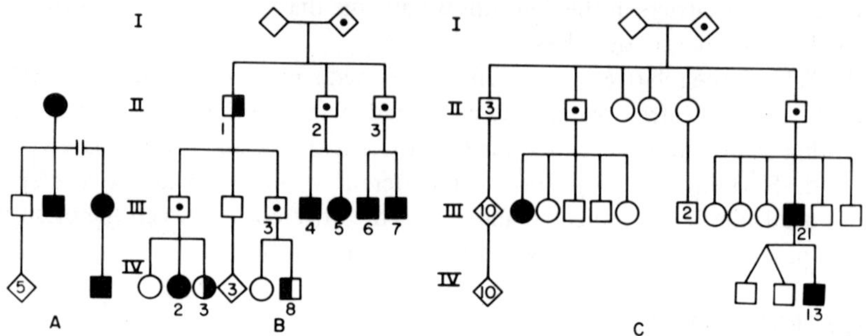

Fig. 1. *Pedigree A* illustrates presumed complete-meiotic mutation in the first affected individual and subsequent dominant transmission of the mutant gene (*Pedigree Ko* from ref. 14). *Pedigree B* illustrates delayed-mitotic mutation in *II-1* (redrawn from ref. 11). *Pedigree C* illustrates possible delayed-meiotic mutation in *III-21* (*Family 41* from ref. 22).

Pedigree B (Fig. 1) is an example of the *Group C* pedigrees which suggest delayed mutation because of the occurrence in collateral relatives. The unilaterally affected grandfather in this family is an example of delayed-mitotic mutation, since he, having unaffected sons but affected grandchildren transmitted to his sons the premutated allele which then underwent (mitotic or meiotic) telomutation in their offspring to produce affected grandchildren. Delayed-meiotic mutation is suggested by occurrence in collateral relatives and subsequent consecutive transmission through one or more generations (Fig. 1, *Pedigree C*).

These types of mutational processes (delayed-mitotic, delayed-meiotic, complete-mitotic, complete-meiotic) cause different proportions of SU, SB, FU and FB cases. Most SU cases apparently result from complete mitotic mutation, but an important minor proportion is due to delayed (meiotic or mitotic) and/or complete-mitotic mutation. Vogel stated that his series of 135 SU parents who produced 21 affected and 290 normal offspring consisted of 120 parents who had only normal children and 15 parents who produced the 21 affected offspring.[10] This suggests that these 15 parents, eg roughly 10% of SU cases, are carriers of the premutant allele each with a risk of 0.37 for producing affected offspring, and that roughly 90% of SU cases each have a negligible risk of producing affected offspring. Sporadic bilaterally affected individuals are presumably due to delayed-meiotic or complete-meiotic mutation. It is possible that a small percentage of SB cases is due to mitotic mutation, but presently the evidence for this is incomplete.

Familial unilateral cases can be due to delayed-meiotic, delayed-mitotic or complete-meiotic mutation. The proportion of FU cases due to delayed-mitotic mutation can be estimated as roughly 60% of total FU cases[5]; those individuals have a recurrence risk similar to that of carriers, namely about 0.37. The other

40% of FU cases have a recurrence risk of 0.5. It is assumed that most, if not all, FB cases are due to either delayed-meiotic or complete-meiotic mutation and that they, therefore, have a 50% risk of having affected offspring.

COUNSELING SITUATIONS

The model of delayed mutation in retinoblastoma may be helpful in specific genetic counseling situations, as, in fact, its predictive power in individual circumstances will validate various aspects as well as the basic idea of the model. It should be noted that in the interpretation of the genetic data on retinoblastoma the implication was tacitly made that all cases of retinoblastoma are assumed to be due to an autosomal dominant mutation (with high or complete penetrance). An important exception to this concerns individuals with chromosomal aberrations such as trisomy 21, trisomy 13, etc, who develop retinoblastoma as a manifestation of the trisomy syndrome. We also consider the 13q deletion syndrome (whether the deletion is interstitial or not) as an example of this category of conditions but we would exclude persons with a normal karyotype in peripheral leukocytes (and fibroblasts) who show chromosome aberrations only in tumor tissue. In general, persons with systemic chromosome aberrations have associated abnormalities, such as mental retardation, shortness of stature, and minor or major malformations. We place all patients with a presumed systemic chromosome aberration in a category different from those more common cases without associated abnormalities and with presumed normal systemic karyotype, and we counsel those families and individuals according to the chromosome aberration.

The counseling in retinoblastoma should not be done unless an extensive family history has been taken, and a complete physical examination has been performed.

Particular attention should be paid to the occurrence of malformations and of tumors for which, in selected cases, a roentgenographic examination may be needed. Of course, both eyes need to be thoroughly examined, and, if possible, it should be noted whether there is a single tumor focus or whether there are multiple foci in the affected eye(s). The age of onset of the tumor(s) and the parental reproductive ages should be stated. Regular follow-up examinations for the development of possible ocular and extraocular tumors are necessary. An affected, enucleated eye should be subjected to further pathologic, histologic, cytogenetic and biochemical investigations by other investigators.

The following remarks concern the cases due to an autosomal dominant mutation. The clinical genetic evaluation of the patient and his family attempts to determine the genotype and to characterize the phenotype of the various family members. Affected individuals have either the mutant or the premutant allele along with the normal allele, and unaffected relatives have either 2 normal alleles or a premutant and a normal allele. Accordingly, members of retinoblastoma families may be classified as normal, affected, or carrier individuals. Normal and affected persons have, respectively, a negligible and a 50% risk to transmit the mutant gene to their offspring. Carrier individuals may transmit the normal, the premutant or the mutant allele to their offspring and empirically they produce 54.5% normal, 36.4% affected and 9.1% carrier offspring (Table 3). This means that among the offspring of carriers 4.5% of carrier offspring are not identified as carriers, that among the unaffected offspring of carriers 21.4% are carriers, and that unaffected sibs of affected persons who have a carrier parent have a 0.21 risk of also being a carrier. The mutant gene we consider fully or nearly fully penetrant, since we are not aware of a single documented instance of decreased penetrance in retinoblastoma; in our opinion, all such postulated cases represent instances of transmission of the premutant allele rather than nonexpressivity of the (fully) mutant allele.

A particular case of retinoblastoma will present phenotypically as sporadic or familial and as unilaterally or bilaterally affected. We consider a case as sporadic, or familial, and unilateral or bilateral, which has undergone a proper genetic, clinical and ophthalmologic evaluation at that point in time; of course, the patient's age is critical, as (s)he may subsequently develop tumor(s) in the other eye or produce affected descendants and thus change from a unilateral to a bilateral and from a sporadic to a familial case. Counseling of sporadic or familial cases most often concerns the recurrence risk for having future affected offspring, grandchildren, sibs or cousins. The situation is somewhat less complicated for bilaterally than for unilaterally affected cases.

Bilateral Cases

Bilaterally affected individuals (sporadic as well as familial cases) are mostly, if not always, considered due to delayed or complete meiotic mutation. They are, therefore, advised of the risk of 50% for affected offspring according to the rules of autosomal dominant transmission. The offspring is likely also to be bilaterally affected, since only 14% of offspring of FB parents were unilaterally affected (Table 3). Complete or almost complete penetrance implies that bilaterally affected individuals are very unlikely to have affected grandchildren, if their offspring are not affected. Again, this holds for sporadic as well as for familial cases. The difficulty in counseling bilaterally affected individuals does not concern their descendants but their sibs. Unaffected parents of a bilaterally affected child could either have the normal gene (and in that case increased paternal reproductive age could indicate the occurrence of a new mutation), or one parent could be a carrier of a premutated allele at the retinoblastoma locus. With a positive family history one would assume the latter condition to be applicable; but in a sporadic case one could not be sure. There are 2 indications that most parents of SB are not carriers: 1) the fact that the mutation at the retinoblastoma locus is more often complete than delayed,[5] and 2) that the empiric risk for sibs of SB cases to be affected is 6.2%.[9] Thus, perhaps about 17% of parents of SB children are carriers. The risk of affected cousins is low in SB cases and in familial cases it depends on the individual pedigree.

Unilateral Cases

In the counseling of unilaterally affected persons the family history and the status of the parents is especially important. FU cases with unaffected parents are considered to be due to delayed-mitotic mutation and to have the same recurrence risk as carriers.[5] FU cases with a bilaterally affected parent are likely to have inherited the mutant and not the premutant allele; these would be counseled similar to the FB cases. For an individual FU case with a unilaterally affected parent it may be difficult to decide whether the premutant or the mutant allele was transmitted, leaving a choice of the risk of affected offspring between 36% vs 50% and a choice of risk of affected grandchildren between virtually zero vs 8% vs 25% depending on whether, respectively, the normal, the premutant or the mutant allele is transmitted to the offspring, eg parent of the grandchild.

Sporadic unilaterally affected cases could have inherited either the normal or the premutated gene. As indicated,[5] one can estimate that perhaps 10% of SU cases are due to delayed-mitotic, delayed-meiotic or complete-meiotic mutation while the large majority appear to be due to complete-mitotic mutation.

Several features of the model of delayed mutation suggest some general means of distinguishing between delayed and complete mutation and, thus, in individual instances between a high and negligible recurrence risk, respectively. One feature is the number of normal sibs, since an increasing number of normal sibs makes it less likely that a parent of a SU child is a carrier of the premutated allele. Possibly, as in SB cases, an increased paternal reproductive age could suggest a new complete-meiotic mutation in a small percentage of SU cases. Another 2 potentially helpful features also need much further investigation, namely, age of onset and multifocal tumor occurrence. We have no conclusive data available but suggest that SU cases due to delayed mutation occur both at an earlier age and are more often multifocal than SU cases due to complete-mitotic mutation. The SU cases due to delayed mutation, of course, have the same risks as carriers, while SU cases due to complete mutation have a negligible risk of affected offspring. The risk of affected relatives other than children differs accordingly.

Empiric Risk Figures

The literature provides some empiric risk figures for certain of the situations outlined above. The most useful data in this respect were published by Briard-Guillemot et al.[9] They found among 165 offspring of unaffected carriers

58.2% normal, 32.3% affected and 11.5% carrier individuals, a distribution which is not significantly different from that shown for carriers in Table 3. The empiric risk of 6.2% for sibs of SB cases[9] to be affected has already been mentioned. Sibs of SU cases have a low empiric risk, namely 0.06%,[9] but they, in turn, have a higher risk of having affected offspring (0.4%) than the sibs of SB cases (no affected offspring known).[9] Briard-Guillemot et al also report figures for familial cases, but they do not differentiate between FU and FB cases.[9] The risk for a sib of a familial case was quoted as 35.7% when the parent of the case was affected and as 12.5% when the parent was not affected. The risk for sibs of familial cases to have affected offspring was 18.8% when the parent of the case was affected but when the parent was not affected no recurrence was seen in 20 instances. Hemmes found none of 253 sibs of 48 sporadic (unilateral and bilateral) cases affected and noted that 76 of these 253 sibs (of 24 patients) had 281 normal children.[20] Gordon reported that for 67 unilaterally affected (sporadic and familial) patients, 3 (1.2%) affected sibs were found among 241, and for 47 bilaterally (sporadic and familial) patients, 9 (8.2%) of 109 sibs were found affected.[21] Schappert-Kimmijser et al found 10 (1.12%) affected of 889 sibs of sporadic cases.[14]

SUMMARY

The genealogic and genetic data on retinoblastoma were reviewed and interpreted according to the model of delayed mutation; then applications of the model to specific situations in genetic counseling were considered. Patients with multiple congenital abnormalities and systemic chromosome aberrations are regarded as belonging to a different category of retinoblastoma cases than the more common patients without such abnormalities. The model of delayed mutation is considered for the latter group of patients.

According to the model, mutation at the retinoblastoma locus can be delayed or complete and can occur during meiotic or mitotic cell division. Genotypically, three clases of individuals can be identified in retinoblastoma families: homozygous normal, heterozygous for the premutated allele, and heterozygous for the (fully) mutated allele; the other possible combinations of individuals have apparently not been observed. There is to date no evidence to suggest incomplete penetrance of the mutant allele, but 14% of individuals who have the mutant gene are "only" unilaterally affected. Carriers produce normal, affected and carrier offspring in the empiric proportion of, respectively, 54.5%, 36.4%, and 9.1%. Most difficulties in genetic counseling arise because affected individuals may have inherited the premutated or the mutated allele and because unaffected individuals may have inherited the normal or the premutated allele. These aspects were considered for individuals presenting as sporadic-unilateral, sporadic-bilateral, familial-unilateral and familial-bilateral cases, and the empiric risk figures for various situations were quoted from the literature.

ACKNOWLEDGMENT

I am grateful to Dr. John M. Opitz for helpful discussion and the critical reading of the manuscript.

REFERENCES

1. Auerbach, C.: A possible case of delayed mutation in man. Ann. Hum. Genet. 20: 266–269, 1956.
2. Opitz, J. M.: Delayed mutation in achondroplasia. In Bergsma, D. (ed.): Part IV. "Skeletal Dysplasias," Birth Defects: Orig. Art. Ser., vol. V, no. 4, White Plains: The National Foundation–March of Dimes, 1969, pp. 20–23.
3. Herrmann, J. and Opitz, J. M.: Delayed mutation as a cause of genetic disease in man: Achondroplasia and the Wiedemann-Beckwith syndrome. In Nichols, W.W. and Miller, R. W. (eds.): "Proc. Workshop on Regulation of Cell Proliferation and Differentiation," 1975. (In press.)
4. Lubinsky, M., Herrmann, J., Kosseff, A. L. and Opitz, J. M.: Autosomal dominant sex-dependent transmission of the Wiedemann-Beckwith syndrome. Lancet 1:932, 1974.
5. Herrmann, J.: Delayed mutation as a cause of retinoblastoma. Submitted for publication to Am. J. Hum. Genet.
6. Auerbach, C.: Chemically induced mosaicism in Drosophila melanogaster. Proc. R. Soc. Edinb. (Biol.) B62:211–221, 1946.
7. Warburg, M.: Retinoblastoma. In Goldberg, M. F. (ed.): "Genetic and Metabolic Eye Disease." Boston: Little, Brown Co., 1974.
8. François, J., Matton, M. T., DeBie, S. et al: Genesis and genetics of retinoblastoma. Ophthalmologica 170:405–425, 1975.
9. Briard-Guillemot, M. L., Bonaiti-Pellié, C., Feingold, J. and Frézal, J.: Étude génétique due rétinoblastome. Humangenetik 24:271–284, 1974.
10. Vogel, F.: Genetic prognosis in retinoblastoma. In Sorsby, A. (ed.): "Modern Trends in Ophthalmology." London: Butterworth, 1967, pp. 34–42.
11. Czeizel, A. and Gárdonyi, J.: Retinoblastoma in Hungary, 1960–1968. Humangenetik 22:153–158, 1974.
12. Jensen, A. D.: Retinoblastoma in Denmark 1943–1958. Acta Ophthalmol. (Kbh.) 43: 821–840, 1965.
13. Tarkhanen, A. and Tuovinen, E.: Retinoblastoma in Finland 1912–1964. Acta Ophthalmol. 49:293–300, 1971.
14. Schappert-Kimmijser, J., Hemmes, G. D. and Nijland, R.: The heredity of retinoblastoma. Ophthalmologica 151:197–213, 1966.
15. Berg, R.: Personal communication.
16. Vogel, F.: Über Genetik und Mutationsrate des Retinoblastoms. Z. Menschl Vererb. U. Konstit.-Lehre 32:308–336, 1954.
17. Falls, H. F. and Neel, J. V.: Genetics of retinoblastoma. Arch. Ophthalmol. 46:367–389, 1951.
18. Smith, S. M. and Sorsby, A.: Retinoblastoma: Some genetic aspects. Ann. Hum. Genet. 23:50–57, 1958.
19. Pellié, C., Briard, M.-L., Feingold, J. and Frézal, J.: Parental age in retinoblastoma. Humangenetik 20:59–62, 1973.
20. Hemmes, G. D.: Untersuchungen nach dem Vorkommen von Glioma retinae bei Verwandten von mit dieser Krankheit Behafteten. Klin. Monatsbl. Augenheilkd. 86: 331–335, 1931.

21. Gordon, H.: Family studies in retinoblastoma. In Bergsma, D. (ed.): "Medical Genetics Today," Birth Defects: Orig. Art. Ser., vol. X, no. 10. Baltimore: The Johns Hopkins University Press for The National Foundation–March of Dimes, 1974, pp. 185–190.

22. Macklin, M. T.: A study of retinoblastoma in Ohio. Am. J. Hum. Genet. 12:1–43, 1960.

23. Böhringer, H. R.: Statistik, Klinik und Genetik der schweizerischen Retinoblastom-fälle (1925–1954). Arch. Klaus-Stift. Vererb.-Forsch. 31:1–16, 1956.

24. Bedford, M. H., Bedotto, C. and Macfaul, P. A.: Retinoblastoma. A study of 139 cases. Br. J. Ophthalmol. 55:19–27, 1971.

25. Czeizel, A., Csósz, L., Gárdonyi, J. et al: Chromosome studies in twelve patients with retinoblastoma. Humangenetik 22:159–166, 1974.

26. Grace, E., Drennan, J., Colver, D and Gordon, R. R.: The 13q-deletion syndrome. J. Med. Genet. 8:351–357, 1971.

27. O'Grady, R. B., Rothstein, T. B. and Romano, P. E.: D-group deletion syndromes and retinoblastoma. Am. J. Ophthalmol. 77:40–45, 1974.

28. Orye, E., Delbeke, M. J. and Vandenbeele, B.: Retinoblastoma and long arm deletion of chromosome 13. Attempts to define the deleted segment. Clin. Genet. 5:457–464, 1974.

29. Wilson, M. G., Towner, J. W. and Fujimoto, A.: Retinoblastoma and D- chromosome deletions. Am. J. Hum. Genet. 25:57–61, 1973.

30. Rethoré, M. O., Saraux, H., Prieur, M. et al: Syndrome 48,XXY, +21 et retinoblastoma. Arch. Fr. Pediatr. 29:533–539, 1972.

31. Herrmann, J., Gilbert, E. F. and Opitz, J. M.: Dysplasia, malformations and cancer especially with respect to the Wiedemann-Beckwith syndrome. In "Proc. Workshop on Regulation of Cell Proliferation and Differentiation." op. cit.

32. Jensen, R. D. and Miller, R. W.: Retinoblastoma: Epidemiologic characteristics. N. Engl. J. Med. 285:307–311, 1971.

33. Kitchin, F. D. and Ellsworth, R. M.: Pleiotropic effects of the gene for retinoblastoma. J. Med. Genet. 11:244–246, 1974.

Genetics of Central Nervous System Tumors

William A. Horton, MD

Tumors of the central nervous system (CNS) are generally not inherited.
There is however, a small group of established disorders in which a CNS tumor
is inherited either singularly or as part of a more diffuse syndrome. In addition,
there are a growing number of reports of familial occurrences of CNS tumors in
which the role of genetic factors is not clear. The purpose of this paper is to
review these 2 categories of CNS tumors.

DISORDERS OF KNOWN INHERITANCE

Of the inherited disorders in which CNS tumors regularly occur, 4 are
phakomatoses: neurofibromatosis, the von Hippel-Lindau syndrome, tuberous
sclerosis, and the multiple nevoid basal cell carcinoma syndrome (Table 1).
All are autosomal dominant traits. The concept of the phakomatoses although
controversial, is useful in discussing the associated tumors. These syndromes
which are thought to reflect disturbed embryologic development are characterized by 3 major types of lesions: the cutaneous manifestations (phakos or
hamarties), the tumorous malformations or stable tumors with little growth
potential (phakomas or hamartomas), and the true tumors in which cellular
proliferation may be marked (phakoblastomas or hamartoblastomas).[1-3] The
tumors under discussion thus represent the third type of lesion involving
the CNS.

The manifestations of the von Recklinghausen syndrome, or neurofibromatosis, result from hyperplasia and neoplasia of neuroectodermal tissue.[4] Based
on location of major involvement, the syndrome can be divided into 3 forms
which tend to remain constant within individual families: a peripheral form
characterized primarily by peripheral nerve and skin lesions; a central form in
which CNS and sympathetic nervous system lesions predominate, and a mixed

Birth Defects: Original Article Series, Volume XII, Number 1, pages 91–97

TABLE 1. Inherited Disorders Manifesting CNS Tumors

Disorder	Genetics	Common CNS Tumors	Uncommon CNS Tumors

Neurofibromatosis	Autosomal dominant	Neurinoma
		Glioma
		  spongioblastoma/
		   glioblastoma
		  astrocytoma
		  ependymoma
		Meningioma
			Gliomatosis cerebri

von Hippel-Lindau syndrome	Autosomal dominant	Hemangioblastoma	Ependymoma Choroid plexus papilloma
Tuberous sclerosis	Autosomal dominant	Giant cell astrocytoma	Glioblastoma multiforme Ependymoma Diffuse gliomatosis Meningioma
Multiple nevoid basal cell carcinoma syndrome	Autosomal dominant		Medulloblastoma
Retinoblastoma	Autosomal dominant	Retinoblastoma	
Multiple endocrine adenomatosis syndrome type I	Autosomal dominant	Pituitary adenoma	
Glioma-polyposis syndrome	Autosomal recessive	Glioblastoma multiforme Medulloblastoma Ependymoma ?	

form.[5] By definition most CNS tumors are found in the latter 2 forms.

The most common tumors arise from the Schwann cell and depending upon the cellular density, degree of neural elements present, encapsulation, and pathologic classification used, have been variously referred to as neurinomas, neurofibromas, neurilemomas, and schwannomas. Intracranially they most often involve cranial nerve VIII, the acoustic neuroma, usually bilaterally.[2] They are seen in 5% of all affected individuals and in a much higher percentage of patients with the central form of the syndrome.[5,6] The average age at diagnosis is 24 years, significantly younger than that of the sporadic unilateral tumor, which is 44 years.[7] Similar tumors occur in a much lower frequency involving cranial nerves V, IX, X, and XI. Schwannomas are also found in the extramedullary portion of the spinal cord most often arising from the dorsal roots in the thoracic and cauda equina regions, where they are often multiple. An intramedullary spinal cord lesion resembling the schwannoma is sometimes observed and has been termed "schwannosis."[8]

The entire spectrum of gliomas, ranging from well-differentiated astrocytomas and ependymomas to diffuse gliosis and gliomatosis, is found. In a large study, 45% of all affected individuals with neurofibromatosis had some form of glioma, and in half of them it was observed at multiple sites.[9] Most of the gliomas fall into the less-differentiated spongioblastoma group and have a predilection for structures deep in the brain.[10] The most prevalent is the optic nerve glioma which occurs in 5–15% of patients, usually in childhood.[4] The astrocytomas are commonly found intracranially as solitary masses, while the ependymomas usually arise in the spinal cord often at multiple sites and frequently coexist with bilateral acoustic neuroma.[2] The rarest form of glial tumor is the so-called gliomatosis cerebri, alternatively termed hyperplastic gliotic foci or disseminated gliosis and gliomatosis. It consists of diffuse gliomatosis involving the cerebral hemispheres and brain stem and produces gradual deterioration of mental function in both children and adults.[8]

Single or multiple meningiomas may develop but are less common; 54% arise intracranially, 4% in the spinal cord and 42% at both sites.[9] Because of their frequent occurrence at multiple sites, the term meningiomatosis is commonly used to describe these tumors, which are also often associated with bilateral acoustic neuroma.[11] Clinically, the meningiomas behave as sporadic tumors but tend to occur at an earlier age.

The CNS hemangioblastoma is the hallmark of the von Hippel-Lindau syndrome. This tumor which has been variously called angioma, hemangioma, and angioreticuloma, is primarily a vascular tumor of mesodermal origin.[12] The most common sites of involvement are the cerebellum in 64% of patients, the retina (retinal angiomatosis) in 50%, the spinal cord in 10%, and the medulla oblongata in 6%.[13] These lesions usually appear in the third and fourth decades, but may range from the first to the seventh. There is a tendency to develop more tumors at different sites with age. Other CNS tumors including cerebral hemangioblastoma, cerebellar ependymoma, and choroid plexus papilloma have been reported, but are rare.[12,14]

Although the most common CNS lesions in tuberous sclerosis are the tubers or nodules of glial proliferation scattered over the surface of the cerebral cortex and ventricles, it has been estimated that from 1–5% of patients have cerebral tumors, usually as children or young adults.[2,4] Histologically the tumors are giant cell astrocytomas and are thought by some to originate from the glial nodules.[15] They occur almost exclusively within the ventricular walls often producing noncommunicating hydrocephalus.[2] Also reported in a much lower frequency are glioblastoma multiforme, ependymoma, diffuse gliomatosis, and meningioma.[4,16]

It is now recognized that medulloblastoma may occur as a feature of the multiple nevoid basal cell carcinoma syndrome. The cerebellar tumor usually occurs before the age of 2 years, and differs little from sporadic medulloblastoma clinically or pathologically.[17]

There are 3 other syndromes, not phakomatoses, in which CNS tumors regularly occur and in which the inheritance has been reasonably defined (Table 1). The bilateral form of retinoblastoma is inherited as an autosomal dominant trait. In addition 5–10% of unilateral retinoblastoma is thought to represent the partially expressed form of this trait.[18] A long arm deletion of chromosome 13 has been noted in several patients with retinoblastoma both with and without associated congenital anomalies.[19] Increased parental age has been noted at time of birth in many of the sporadic cases.[20] Although the pituitary adenoma of multiple endocrine adenomatosis type I (MEA-I) is not strictly a CNS tumor, this autosomal dominant disorder is included because of its location. As many as 65% of patients with the syndrome develop pituitary adenomas, usually chromophobic or less frequently eosinophilic adenomas.[21] Other families in which pituitary adenomas are associated with acromegaly or the amenorrhea/galactorrhea syndrome but without other evidence of MEA-I have been reported, but controversy exists as to whether or not these cases represent partial forms of MEA-I.[22] The association of gliomas and polyposis of the colon has been noted in at least 3 families, in which the inheritance has been consistent with an autosomal recessive pattern. In one of the families, medulloblastoma was noted in one patient, and in another family a second cousin had a posterior fossa ependymoma.[23–25]

FAMILIAL AGGREGATION OF CNS TUMORS

In recent years there have been a number of reports of familial aggregations of CNS tumors (Table 2). In general, family members have manifested tumors which were very similar histologically as well as in biologic behavior. Most

TABLE 2. CNS Tumors Which Aggregate in Families

Glioma
    gliomatosis-glioblastomatosis*
    astrocytoma
    ependymoma
    oligodendroglioma
Meningioma
Medulloblastoma

*Poorly differentiated and diffuse glioma

families have had tumors of the glioma group, the majority at the more malignant end of the glioma spectrum. These families have been grouped into a broad category termed familial gliomatosis-glioblastomatosis. In general, the tumors are composed of immature poorly differentiated cells lying deep in the brain in the region of the ventricular germinal centers. They grow by infiltration and involve particularly the frontal, temporal, parietooccipital regions and corpus callosum.[1] This group of tumors has been reported in sibs, 2 consecutive generations, and in mono- and dizygotic twins in which concordance for the tumor has been variable.[26-31] Usually the tumors are present during adulthood but they have been reported during childhood.[32]

Similar family aggregations of more differentiated gliomas, the astrocytomas, ependymomas, oligodendrogliomas have been noted.[27,33-35] The tumors differ little from their sporadic counterparts except for a younger age at onset in the familial cases.

Less commonly, meningiomas have been reported in sibs, 2 consecutive generations, and in one pair of concordant monozygotic twins.[36-38] Medulloblastoma has been described in sibs, half sibs, and monozygotic twins.[27,39,40]

In the first category of established disorders, the role of genetic factors is relatively clear. All are transmitted in an autosomal dominant manner except the glioma-polyposis syndrome, which appears to show autosomal recessive inheritance. In the second category, however, the importance of these factors is far from clear. Studies showing a greater-than-expected frequency of major CNS malformations in the families with tumors have suggested that errors in early CNS development may serve as a basis for CNS tumor formation in later life, likening these tumors to those that occur in the phakomatoses.[41,42] Another recent study, however, has shown no such correlation.[43] Similarily, large statistical studies to evaluate the risk of CNS tumor in relatives of patients with such tumors, have yielded conflicting results.[34,44] Twin studies are too few in number to draw any conclusions. The significance of the partial chromosome deletion in some cases of retinoblastoma is not clear. Thus, although genetic factors are likely implicated, the extent and mechanisms involved must await further investigation.

CONCLUSION

Although central nervous system tumors are generally not inherited, there are 7 presently recognized genetic disorders, 4 of which are phakomatoses, in which such tumors regularly occur. In addition, certain tumors, mainly gliomas, do occasionally aggregate within families.

REFERENCES

1. Koch, G.: Genetic aspect of the phakomatoses. In Vinken, P. J. and Bruyn, G. W. (eds.): Handbook of Clinical Neurology: The Phakomatoses. New York: American Elsevier Publishing Co., Inc., 1972, pp. 488–561.
2. de Recondo, J. and Haguenau, M.: Neuropathologic survey of the phakomatoses and allied disorders. In Vinken, P. J. and Bruyn, G. W. (eds.): Ibid. pp. 19–101.
3. Wechsler, W.: Old and new concepts of oncogenesis in the nervous system of man and animals. Prog. Exp. Tumor Res. 17:219–278, 1972.
4. Aita, J. A.: Genetic aspects of tumors of the nervous system. Nebr. Med. J. 53: 121–124, 1968.
5. Allen, J. C., Eldridge, R. and Young, D.: Early-onset acoustic neuroma: Genetic, clinical and nosologic aspects. In Bergsma, D. (ed): Medical Genetics Today, Birth Defects: Orig. Art. Ser., vol. X, no. 10. Baltimore: The Johns Hopkins University Press for The National Foundation–March of Dimes, 1974, pp. 171–184.
6. Crowe, F. W., Schull, W. J. and Neel, J. V.: A Clinical, Pathological and Genetic Study of Multiple Neurofibromatosis. Springfield: Charles C Thomas, 1956.
7. Edwards, C. H. and Paterson, J. H.: A review of the symptoms and signs of acoustic neurofibromatosis. Brain 74:144–190, 1951.
8. Canale, D. J. and Bebin, J.: von Recklinghausen disease of the nervous system. In Vinken, P. J. and Bruyn, G. W. (eds.): op. cit. pp. 132–163.
9. Rodriguez, H. A. and Berthrong, M.: Multiple primary intracranial tumors in von Recklinghausen's neurofibromatosis. Arch. Neurol. 14:467–475, 1966.
10. Zulch, K. J.: Le spongioblastome et la maladie de Recklinghausen. In Michaux, L. and Feld, M. (eds.): Les Phakomatoses Cérébrales, Paris: SPEI, 1963.
11. Rovine, B. W. and Mulford, E. H.: Bilateral acoustic neurinomas with multiple meningiomas. Neurology (Minneap.) 10:323–324, 1960.
12. Melmon, K. L. and Rosen, S. W.: Lindau's disease: Review of the literature and study of a large kindred. Am. J. Med. 36:595–617, 1964.
13. Horton, W. A.: Unpublished data.
14. Lauritsen, J. G.: Lindau's disease: A study of one family through six generations. Acta Chir. Scand. 139:482–486, 1973.
15. Russell, D. S. and Rubenstein, L. J.: Pathology of Tumors of the Nervous System. 2nd Ed. London: Edward Arnold, Ltd., 1963.
16. Donegani, G., Grattarola, F. R. and Wildi, E.: Tuberous sclerosis. Bourneville disease. In Vinken, P. J. and Bruyn, G. W. (eds.): op. cit. pp. 340–399.
17. Gorlin, R. J. and Sedano, H. O.: Multiple nevoid basal cell carcinoma syndrome. In Vinken, P. J. and Bruyn, G. W. (eds.): op. cit. pp. 455–473.
18. Sorsby, A.: Bilateral retinoblastoma: A dominantly inherited affection. Br. Med. J. 2: 580–583, 1972.
19. Niebuhr, E. and Ottosen, J.: Ring chromosome D (13) associated with multiple congenital malformations. Ann. Genet. 16:157–166, 1973.
20. Fraser, G. R. and Friedman, A. I.: Retinoblastoma. In The Causes of Blindness in

Childhood. Baltimore: The Johns Hopkins University Press, 1967, p. 11.

21. Ballard, H.S., Frame, B. and Hartsock, R. J.: Familial multiple endocrine adenoma-peptic ulcer complex. Medicine 43:481, 1964.

22. Rimoin, D. L. and Schimke, R. N.: Genetic Disorders of the Endocrine Glands. St. Louis: C. V. Mosby Co., 1971, pp. 52–55.

23. Turcot, J., Depres, J. P. and Pierre, F. S.: Malignant tumors of the central nervous system associated with familial polyposis of the colon. Dis. Colon Rectum 2:465–468, 1959.

24. Baughman, F. A., List, C. F., Williams, J. R. et al: The glioma-polyposis syndrome. N. Engl. J. Med. 281:1345–1346, 1969.

25. McKusick, V. A.: Mendelian Inheritance in Man. 3rd Ed., Baltimore: The Johns Hopkins University Press, 1971, p. 531.

26. Armstrong, R. M. and Hanson, C. W.: Familial gliomas. Neurology 19:1061–1063, 1969.

27. Kjellin, K., Muller, R. and Anstrom, K. E.: The occurrence of brain tumors in several members of a family. J. Neuropathol. Exp. Neurol. 19:528–537, 1960.

28. Koch, G.: Phakomatosen. In Becker, P. E. (ed.) Humangenetik. Krankheiten des Nervensystems. Stuttgart: G. Thieme, 1966, vol. 5, no. 1, pp. 34–111.

29. Koch, G.: Ergebnisse aus der Nachuntersuchung der Berliner Zwillingsserie nach 20–25 Jahren (vorlaufige Ergebnisse). Acta Genet (Basel) 7:47–52, 1957.

30. MacFarland, J. and Meade, T. S.: The genetic origins of tumors supported by their simultaneous and symmetrical occurrence in homologous twins. Am. J. Med. Sci. 184:66–80, 1932.

31. Hauge, M. and Harvald, B.: Genetics in intracranial tumors. Acta Genetica et Statistica Medica 7:537–591, 1957.

32. Fairburn, B. and Urich, H.: Malignant gliomas occurring in identical twins. J. Neurol. Neurosurg. Psychiatry 34:718–722, 1971.

33. Isamat, F., Miranda, M. A., Bartumeus, F. and Prat, J.: Genetic implications of familial brain tumors. J. Neurosurg. 41:573–575, 1974.

34. Metzel, E.: Betrachtungen zur Genetik der familiären Gliome. Acta Genet. Med. Gemellol. (Roma) 13:124, 1964.

35. Parkinson, D. and Hall, C. W.: Oligodendrogliomas. Simultaneous appearance in frontal lobes of siblings. J. Neurosurg. 19:424–426, 1962.

36. Joynt, R. J. and Perret, G. E.: Familial meningiomas. J. Neurol. Neurosurg. Psychiatry 28:163–164, 1965.

37. Sahar, A.: Familial occurrence of meningiomas. J. Neurosurg. 23:444–445, 1965.

38. Sedzimir, C. B., Frazer, A. K. and Roberts, J. R.: Cranial and spinal meningiomas in a pair of identical twin boys. J. Neurol. Neurosurg. Psychiatry 36:368–376, 1973.

39. Belamaric, J. and Chau, A. S.: Medulloblastoma in newborn sisters. J. Neurosurg. 30:76–79, 1969.

40. Griepentrog, F. and Pauly, H.: Intra-und extrakranielle, frühmanifeste Medulloblastome bei erbgleichen Zwillingen. Zentralbl. Neurochir. 17:129–140, 1957.

41. van der Wiel, H. J.: Inheritance of Glioma: The Genetic Aspects of Cerebral Glioma and Its Relation to Status Dysraphicus. Amsterdam: Elsevier Publishing Co., Inc., 1960, p. 275.

42. Miller, R. W.: Relation between cancer and congenital defects in man. N. Engl. J. Med. 275:87–93, 1966.

43. De Weerdt, C. J. and Schut, T.: Some aspects of heredity of brain tumors. Psychiatr. Neurol. Neurochir. 75:293–298, 1972.

44. Hauge, M. and Harvald, B.: Studies in the etiology of intracranial tumors. Acta Psychiatr. Scand. 35:163–170, 1960.

Genetic Factors in Pulmonary Neoplasms

John J. Mulvihill, MD

The epidemic of lung cancer continues. In 1970, about 80,000 people developed lung cancer in the United States.[1]

Conventional approaches to understanding the etiology of lung cancer have with profit focused on environmental agents.[2] Efforts to identify and control human carcinogens have been most successful with respect to the hazards of occupational inhalants associated with radioactive ores, mustard gas, asbestos, nickel, chromates, arsenic, and certain petrochemicals. In contrast, the commonest human carcinogen in the general population, tobacco smoke, is poorly characterized regarding carcinogenic mechanisms and poorly controlled through public education. Pending development of less hazardous cigarettes and advances in motivational research, it is timely to identify host factors that alter susceptibility to known respiratory carcinogens. An appreciation of genetic factors may help occupational health workers to identify individuals at high risk and may contribute to further knowledge of carcinogenesis.

DEMOGRAPHIC VARIABLES

Standard epidemiologic data give little clue to host-related factors.[3] The changing incidence of lung cancer in this century — a 20-fold increase for males in 30 years — certainly cannot be accounted for by large changes in mutation rates or gene pools. Evolving X-linked traits do not explain the rapidly changing sex ratio — peaking at 6.8 males to 1 female case in 1960. Rather, they are well explained by trends in tobacco use, assuming a 30-year induction period.[4] Within the U.S., racial differences await explanation. Compared to whites, lung cancer mortality is accelerating more rapidly in blacks[5] and is lower in American Indians[6] and higher in Americans of Mexican[7] and Chinese extraction.[8]

Birth Defects: Original Article Series, Volume XII, Number 1, pages 99—111

The geographic distribution of lung cancer in the U.S. suggests variations from occupational exposures and not by ethnic groups, except for a concentration in southern Louisana, where inbreeding is conspicuous.[9] Striking variations occur worldwide: There is an 8-fold range in incidence among males and the sex ratio varies markedly with relatively fewer cases in Israel and Ireland.[10] These differences could arise from environmental and/or genetic factors, which can sometimes be distinguished by studying the cancer experience of migrants. For lung cancer, the observations are inconclusive: The migrant rates seem intermediate between the rates in their former and new countries.[11] However, among Chinese, the rate is high both in the Orient and the U.S.[8] An additional peculiarity of the Chinese is the predominance of adenocarcinoma of the lung in Hong Kong, a relatively infrequent cell type.[12]

Age relates strongly to certain cell types. Bronchogenic carcinoma is seldom seen in children and young adults.[13] The Third National Cancer Survey, a 10% sample of the U.S. population, 1969–1971, recorded no cases of primary lung tumors under age 20.[14] In 9 years, the U.S. Childhood Cancer Mortality Registry ascertained only 60 primary lung tumors under age 20. There were no carcinomas under age 5 years when prenatal origins may be suspected — all were sarcomas, teratomas, and hemangiomas.[15]

Studies of twins have not shown a genetic factor because of inadequate numbers of cases; however, one study of 10,945 twin pairs demonstrated the influence of smoking on lung cancer.[16]

EMPIRIC FAMILIAL RISK

Where demography has failed, a more refined tool, the case-control study, has shown a significant familial factor, which could be environmental and genetic. Tokuhata and Lilienfeld found 2.4 to 2.7 times more lung cancer among relatives of lung cancer patients than among relatives of controls.[17, 18] The familial factor was more evident among nonsmokers than among smokers. Conversely, the effect of smoking was less evident among case relatives (who had the familial tendency already) than among control relatives. The familial and smoking effects were synergistic (Fig. 1). These pioneer studies were well done: Controls were matched by sex, age, race, and residence; spouse controls were included; and diagnoses were histologically confirmed. In contrast, the only subsequent study was much smaller and showed no familial tendency.[19]

The data of Tokuhata and Lilienfeld were not analyzed by histologic cell type. Like other common cancers that show a 3-fold recurrence risk in families (eg breast, stomach, and colon),[20] lung cancer is a heterogeneous disease with various cell types and suspected etiologic agents. Study of homogeneous subgroups of lung cancer patients might reveal, for certain rare cell types, strong genetic factors that are undetectable when all cell types are combined. Thus,

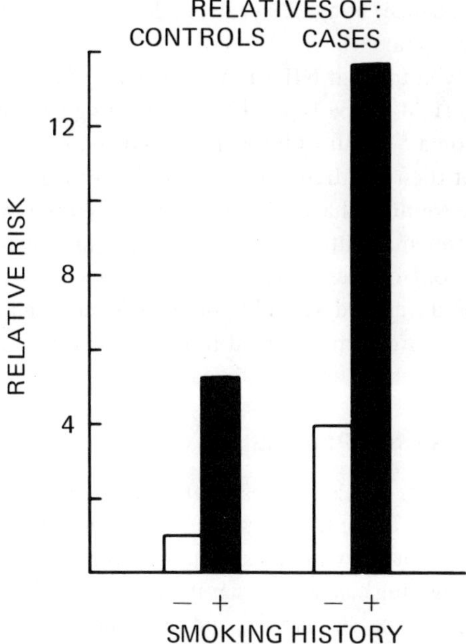

Fig. 1. Risk of lung cancer in relatives of lung cancer cases and controls, by history of smoking.[17] Risk of lung cancer among nonsmoking relatives of controls equals one.

for breast cancer in general, case-control studies have revealed a 3-fold excess in families, but Anderson has identified small subgroups of women with a 47-fold risk in a pattern suggesting a mendelian dominant trait.[21]

PEDIGREE ANALYSIS

Two striking sibships with squamous cell carcinoma of the lung have been reported. In the first, 3 of 7 brothers and one sister developed tumors in their 50s over a period of 2 years.[22] One brother had worked in a copper smelter; the other had been exposed to chromium fumes. In the second sibship, squamous cell carcinoma of the bronchus occurred almost simultaneously in 3 brothers, ages 56−66 years.[23] Two of 3 sisters had cancer of other sites. In both families, the patients with lung cancer had been heavy smokers, a trait well-demonstrated to have strong familial tendency in both twin and case-control studies.[16,17]

Lung cancer is occasionally seen in families that seem to have an excess of tumors of diverse cell types. It appears in pedigrees with excessive ovarian and breast cancers.[24] In one family with the familial soft-tissue sarcoma-breast cancer syndrome,[25] a father developed alveolar cell carcinoma of the lung, his

daughter had breast cancer at age 28 years, and her son died from a rhabdomyosarcoma at age 2 years.

In another family studied at NIH, a 70-year-old proband with Waldenström
macroglobulinemia (IgM kappa type) developed a lung mass that proved to be
alveolar cell carcinoma.[26] Four of his 8 sibs also had a lymphoproliferative disorder, as did one of their children. At initial study, 4 of the offspring who were
clinically well were found to have impaired in vitro lymphocyte transformation
in response to phytohemagglutinin, and 3 of these had polyclonal elevations in
IgM. Subsequently, one of these developed pulmonary adenocarcinoma and her
3-year-old grandson developed acute lymphoblastic leukemia. Thus, a rare type
of lung cancer, adenocarcinoma, seemed to have a genetic and immunologic
basis in a family with clinical and subclinical lymphoproliferative disorders.

MULTIPLE PRIMARY NEOPLASMS

This family and others[24] also suggest that lung cancer may occur as a second
primary neoplasm more often than expected by chance alone. Among all
patients with multiple primary neoplasms in the Connecticut Tumor Registry,[27]
the risk of developing lung cancer was significantly elevated in men with cancer
of the lip, mouth, pharynx, and larynx, and in women with cervical cancer. For
men, the risk may be attributed to continued use of tobacco which may also contribute to the risk in both sexes of later bladder cancer. (The converse strengthens
this possibility: Lung cancer patients have a significant risk for subsequently
developing cancer of the mouth and upper respiratory tract.[28]) Finally, lung
cancer was reported in asssociation with antimetabolite therapy for malignancy[29]
and psoriasis.[30]

IMMUNE FACTORS

Besides these case reports, scattered evidence is accumulating that relates immune factors to the genesis of some lung tumors. First, in a large series of lung
cancer patients, T-lymphocyte levels were depressed at the time of diagnosis.[31]
(But, in 42 patients with multiple primary neoplasms, including 21 with lung
cancer, the numbers of T lymphocytes and distribution of HL-A types were
normal.[32]) Second, uranium miners, known to be at high risk for radiogenic
lung tumors, had normal immunoglobulin levels at the time of employment,
but these fell after one year and remained low even 10 years later.[33] Third, lung
cancer has occurred in 8 renal transplant recipients on immunosuppression, compared to 1.8 expected.[34] Fourth, intensive drug and radiation therapy for extra-
pulmonary malignancy regularly produces atypia of alveolar linings.[35] Finally,
certain disorders with immunologic abnormalities may be associated with lung
cancer, such as dermatomyositis, sarcoidosis, and scleroderma. A strong
heritable tendency has been observed in each of these conditions, except

dermatomyositis, which, in fact, seems to be a paraneoplastic manifestation of lung cancer and not a disease predisposing to it.[36] In 2544 patients with sarcoidosis studied in 10 years, 9 lung tumors were seen compared to 2.8 expected.[37] The cell types were 3 squamous cell, 3 anaplastic small cell, one alveolar cell, one solid adenocarcinoma, and one unknown.[38]

By 1975, over 25 patients with scleroderma (progressive systemic sclerosis) were reported with alveolar cell carcinoma of the lung.[39] Striking features of the association are the 7:1 female-to-male ratio (compared to 2–3:1 for scleroderma in general) and positive correlation with the intensity of interstitial pulmonary fibrosis. The observed progression of fibrosis to lung cancer in scleroderma is likely to be a common route by which various disorders predispose to cancer especially alveolar cell carcinoma.[40] This concept of pathogenesis, similar to that suggested for hepatocellular carcinoma following cirrhosis, unites under the rubric of "scar carcinoma" such diverse pneumonic processes as pulmonary infarction, rheumatic mitral valvular heart disease, and desquamative interstitial pneumonia. In these conditions, intermediary alveolar metaplasia and benign adenomatosis are frequent autopsy findings, and the tumors are thought to be multifocal in origin. (Incidentally, tuberculous patients probably have no excess of lung cancer[41–43] despite earlier reports to the contrary.[41])

Besides the immunologic defects, the finding of excessive chromosomal breaks in peripheral blood and bone marrow of patients with scleroderma supports its malignant potential.[44] Breaks were seen also when cells from normal controls were preincubated in serum from affected patients. Although another study related the breaks to cyclophosphamide therapy,[45] scleroderma may join the group of chromosomal fragility syndromes which predispose to malignancy.

ANTECEDENT HERITABLE LUNG DISEASE

Scleroderma may explain certain familial aggregations of lung tumors, such as the sisters reported by Petitjean,[46] one of whom had alveolar cell carcinoma. Another sibship of 2 brothers with alveolar cell carcinoma was probably explained by the concomitant familial diffuse interstitial pulmonary fibrosis (present also in a cousin without tumor).[47] An autosomal dominant form of congenital cystic disease of the lung (familial fibrocystic pulmonary dysplasia), indistinguishable from Hamman-Rich syndrome except by its chronicity and inheritance, accounted for lung cancer in 2 brothers[48] and for sporadic lung tumors in members of other affected families.[49, 50]

Other autosomal dominant traits have interstitial pulmonary fibrosis as an occasional feature and could be associated with lung cancer, although there are no reports to my knowledge. These syndromes include certain of the phakomatoses (neurofibromatosis, tuberous sclerosis, and Von Hippel-Lindau disease[51]), the Marfan syndrome,[52] and familial pulmonary alveolar microlithiasis.[53]

As for autosomal recessive traits, the occurrence of pulmonary liposarcoma in one of 4 sisters with congenital adrenal hyperplasia is probably a coincidence,[54] but may be iatrogenic, since hyperadrenocorticism can cause large mediastinal lipomas.[55] Multiple leiomyomata, sometimes a recessive trait when it affects the skin,[56] can also involve the lungs.[57] A 52-year-old man was reported with the Kartagener syndrome and bronchogenic carcinoma,[58] again probably fortuitous despite the presence of immunodeficiency and pulmonary malformations which may predispose to lung cancer in other disorders.

In one Swedish family, autosomal dominant inheritance of pulmonary interstitial fibrosis and an abnormal hemogloblin (Malmö) was associated with anaplastic small cell carcinoma.[59] The authors suggest 2 closely linked genes to account for the inheritance pattern because 2 of the 7 members with abnormal chest radiographs lacked hemoglobin Malmö. An American family with hemoglobin Malmö had no pulmonary disorder.[60]

GENETIC MARKERS, INCLUDING ARYL HYDROCARBON HYDROXYLASE

A more public and controversial marker is the inducibility of aryl hydrocarbon hydroxylase (AHH).[61] In experimental systems, polycyclic hydrocarbons are potent carcinogens; they are also found in cigarette smoke. On closer look, the active carcinogen is not the parent compound; certain intermediate metabolites, often epoxides that intercalate with DNA, are potent mutagens and carcinogens and are produced by bronchial mucosa in tissue culture.[62] AHH represents a multiple component enzyme system that catalyzes endogenous and exogenous lipid-like molecules to more polar ones for better elimination. It is found in human lungs, specifically in alveolar macrophages, in peripheral monocytes,[63] and in fact in most organs. In man, cigarette smoking can induce sustained elevation of AHH.[64] In mice, variation in inducibility is present in many but not all inbred strains, in some as an autosomal dominant, in others as a codominant trait.[65]

Relating AHH to human lung cancer, the Kellermans and C. R. Shaw of the M. D. Anderson Hospital made 2 simple but stunning observations. First, AHH inducibility in man seemed to be controlled by a single locus with 2 alleles.[66] Second, in a series of patients with lung cancer, 96% (compared to 55% in controls) had high or intermediate levels of inducibility; low levels were found in 4% of lung cancer patients but in 45% of controls.[67]

For several reasons, the early promise of these findings has faded. First, simple mendelian inheritance is unlikely in man because AHH is not one but several enzymes and because codominance occurs in inbred mice. Second, evidence for one locus with 2 alleles comes from a frequency distribution of inducibility that was said to have 3 modes,[66] but the small number of cases makes the interpretation tenuous. Third, the Houston assay depended on lymphocytes stimulated by mitogens and might not reflect the metabolic activity of bronchial mucosa. Furthermore, T-cell function is depressed in many lung cancer patients,[31] who would thus be unavailable for the Houston assay because their lymphocytes do not transform. In mice, lymphocytic transformability itself appears to be a heritable trait.[68] Finally, one fourth of the 50 Houston patients had adenocarcinoma, a cell type not clearly related to smoking.

Certainly a biochemical or genetic marker of cancer susceptibility would be a welcome advance. Although the relation of AHH inducibility to human lung cancer may be debatable, there is no better candidate trait. Genetic deficiency of α_1-antitrypsin predisposes to panlobular emphysema[69] and lung cancer occurs to excess in patients with emphysema, but of the opposite variety, namely centrilobular.[70] In any case, α_1-antitrypsin levels are increased in lung cancer patients.[71] As for other genetic markers, Terasaki reported a significant excess of HL-A haplotype A1 and A7.[72] Blood group B has been associated with adenocarcinoma, and group O with undifferentiated cancer of the lung in males.[73]

Although chromosomal analysis of lung tumor tissue shows hyperploidy, it has not been well studied.[74] A brief case report of a patient with the Klinefelter syndrome and XY/XXY mosaicism is much cited because the aneuploid cell line showed excessive transformability with the oncogenic SV40; the patient also had lung cancer.[75]

ANIMAL MODELS

Several inbred strains of mice readily develop lung tumors, spontaneously and in response to chemicals.[76,77] Heston estimates that 6 different loci relate to susceptibility to chemically-induced tumors.[78] When urethan is administered to pregnant mice, depending upon the time of injection, the offspring have either pulmonary adenomas at birth or later in life, or malformations of the skeleton, liver, and lung.[79] The spectrum of transplacental carcinogenesis also extends to the F_2 generation, that is, those whose parents had been exposed in utero.[80]

Comparative pathology of pulmonary tumors in domestic animals might offer clues to etiology; for, they frequently share man's environment. For example, only dogs seem to have an appreciable frequency of bronchogenic carcinoma and, of all animals, share man's niche most closely.[81] In a microepidemic of lung cancer among ducks, geese, and swan at the Philadelphia zoo, attributed to airborne carcinogens, genetic factors may have played a role because the highest rates occurred in just 2 breeds, the shoveler and redhead ducks.[82] Of

462,305 domestic animals reported by 13 North American veterinary school clinics to the National Cancer Institute,[83] 126 lung carcinomas were seen (107 canine, 9 feline, 5 bovine, 2 equine, and 3 other small animal species).[84] The only breed that had any excess risk was the Weimaraner with 8 cases compared to 0.4 expected.

Worldwide, alveolar cell carcinoma (jaagsiekte*) is very common in certain herds of sheep.[81] Even within one breed, only selected flocks are affected, suggesting with other clues, an infectious etiology. Transmission by cell-free extracts of neoplastic lungs and strong morphologic and biochemical evidence point to a murine C-type RNA virus.[85]

CONCLUSIONS

Genetic heterogeneity, the leitmotif of the Birth Defects Conferences[86] must be recognized in lung cancer as well. In bronchogenic carcinoma, for example, cigarette smoking is the most important etiologic factor and there is little evidence for inherited influences. On the other hand, numerous peculiarities of adenocarcinoma and alveolar cell carcinoma suggest familial factors: they are poorly related to smoking, they are found in families with acquired immune diseases or heritable disorders of the lung, especially those associated with pulmonary interstitial fibrosis and scleroderma, and they occur as an autosomal dominant trait in mice. Alveolar cell carcinoma has also been identified as a viral disease in sheep.

For other unusual cell types, genetic factors may emerge when sufficient cases are assembled. The syndromes of multiple endocrine adenomatosis (MEA), archetypes of the concept of "apudoma"[87] and "neurocristopathy,"[88] have pulmonary neoplasms, such as bronchial mucosal neuroma in MEA III and bronchial carcinoid in MEA I (Wermer syndrome).[89] Carcinoid alone can be an autosomal dominant trait and shares many histologic, histochemical, and endocrinologic features with oat-cell carcinoma.[90]

In searching out additional genetic factors, the area to examine may be the interaction of known environmental carcinogens with susceptible genotypes.[91] This field might be termed "ecogenetics," a word already in use in general genetics to apply to the long-term effects of the environment on the genome, but it may tolerate a special use in medical genetics. By analogy to pharmacogenetics, the study of variations in the response to drugs, clinical ecogenetics could be the study of variations in the response to environmental agents in general. One challenge in clinical ecogenetics might be the development of the means for screening potential employees for abnormal

---

*The name is said to derive from the African for "hunt sickness," because the afflicted sheep are dyspneic as normal sheep would be from running in a hunt.

genotypes that predispose them to disease following occupational exposures that are harmless to normal genotypes.

REFERENCES

1. Cutler, S. J., Scotto, J., Devesa, S. S. and Connelly, R. R.: Third National Cancer Survey – An overview of available information. J. Natl. Cancer Inst. 53:1565–1575, 1974.
2. Fraumeni, J. F., Jr.: Chemicals in the induction of respiratory tract tumors. In "Cancer Epidemiology, Environmental Factors." Proc. XI International Cancer Congress. Amsterdam: Excerpta Medica, 1974, vol. 3, pp. 327–335.
3. Schneiderman, M. A. and Levin, D. L.: Trends in lung cancer: Mortality, incidence, diagnosis, treatment, smoking and urbanization. Cancer 30:1320–1325, 1972.
4. Burbank, F.: U.S. lung cancer death rates begin to rise proportionately more rapidly for females than for males: A dose-response effect? J. Chronic Dis. 25:473–479, 1972.
5. Burbank, F. and Fraumeni, J. F., Jr.: U.S. cancer mortality: Nonwhite predominance. J. Natl. Cancer Inst. 49:649–659, 1972.
6. Creagan, E. T. and Fraumeni, J. F., Jr: Cancer mortaility among American Indians, 1950–67. J. Natl. Cancer Inst. 49:959–967, 1972.
7. Buell, P. E., Mendez, W. M. and Dunn, J. E., Jr.: Cancer of the lung among Mexican immigrant women in California. Cancer 22:186–192, 1968.
8. Fraumeni, J. F., Jr. and Mason, T. J.: Cancer mortality among Chinese Americans, 1950–69. J. Natl. Cancer Inst. 52:659–665, 1974.
9. Mason, T. J., McKay, F. W., Hoover, R. et al: "Atlas of Cancer Mortality for U.S. Counties: 1950–1969." DHEW Publ. No. (NIH) 75–780. Wash. D. C.: U.S. Govt. Printing Office, 1975.
10. Segi, M., Kurihara, M. and Matsuyama, T.: "Cancer Mortality for Selected Sites in 24 Countries. No. 5. (1964–1965)." Sendai: Tohoku University School of Medicine, 1969.
11. Lilienfeld, A. M., Levin, M. L. and Kessler, I. I.: "Cancer in the United States." Cambridge: Harvard University Press, 1972.
12. Belamaric, J.: Malignant tumors in Chinese: A report based on biopsy and autopsy material from Chinese in Hong Kong. Int. J. Cancer 4:560–573, 1969.
13. Niitu, Y., Kubota, H., Hasegawa, S. et al: Lung cancer (squamous cell carcinoma) in adolescence. Am. J. Dis. Child. 127:108–111, 1974.
14. Young, J. L., Jr. and Miller, R. W.: Incidence of malignant tumors in U.S. children. J. Pediatr. 86:254–258, 1975.
15. Miller, R.W.: Unpublished data.
16. Cederlöf, R., Floderus, B. and Friberg, L.: Cancer in MZ and DZ twins. Acta Genet. Med. Gemellol. (Roma) 19:69–74, 1970.
17. Tokuhata, G. K. and Lilienfeld, A. M.: Familial aggregation of lung cancer in humans. J. Natl. Cancer Inst. 30:289–312, 1963.
18. Tokuhata, G. K. and Lilienfeld, A. M.: Familial aggregation of lung cancer among hospital patients. Public Health Report 78:277–283, 1963.
19. Asal, N. R. and Anderson, P. S., Jr.: The etiology of lung cancer in Northeastern Oklahoma. Health Service Report 87:743–748, 1972.
20. Anderson, D. E.: Familial susceptibility. In Fraumeni, J. F., Jr. (ed.): "Persons at High Risk of Cancer: An Approach to Cancer Etiology and Control." New York: Academic Press. (In press.)
21. Anderson, D. E.: Genetic study of breast cancer: Identification of a high risk group. Cancer 34:1090–1097, 1974.

22. Brisman, R., Baker, R. R., Elkins, R. and Hartmann, W. H.: Carcinoma of lung in four siblings. Cancer 20:2048–2053, 1967.

23. Nagy, I.: Zur Beobachtung von Brochialkarzinomen bei drei Brüdern. Prax. Pneumol. 22:718–723, 1968.

24. Lynch, H. T. and Krush, A. J.: Carcinoma of the breast and ovary in three families. Surg. Gynecol. Obstet. 133:644–648, 1971.

25. Li, F. P. and Fraumeni, J. F., Jr.: Soft-tissue sarcomas, breast cancer, and other neoplasms: A familial syndrome? Ann. Intern. Med. 71:747–752, 1969.

26. Fraumeni, J. F., Jr., Wertelecki, W., Blattner, W. A. et al: Varied manifestations of a familial lymphoproliferative disorder. Am. J. Med. 59:145–151, 1975.

27. Schoenberg, B. S.: "Multiple Primary Malignancies: The Connecticut Experience." New York: Springer-Verlag. (In press.)

28. Berg, J. W., Schottenfeld, D. and Ritter, F.: Incidence of multiple primary cancers. III. Cancers of the respiratory and upper digestive system as multiple primary cancers. J. Natl. Cancer Inst. 44:263–274, 1970.

29. Canellos, G. P., Arseneau, J. C., DeVita, V. T. et al: Second malignancies complicating Hodgkin's disease in remission. Lancet 1:947–949, 1975.

30. Bailin, P. L., Tindall, J. P., Roenigk, H. H. and Hogan, M. D.: Is methotrexate therapy for psoriasis carcinogenic? JAMA 232:359–362, 1975.

31. Dellon, A. L., Potvin, C. and Chretien, P. B.: Thymus-dependent lymphocyte levels in bronchogenic carcinoma: Correlations with histology, clinical stage, and clinical course after surgical treatment. Cancer 35:687–694, 1975.

32. Dellon, A. L., Chretien, P. B., Potvin, C. and Rogentine, G. N., Jr.: Multiple primary malignant neoplasms. A search for an immunogenetic basis. Arch. Surg. 110:156–160, 1975.

33. Andrlíková, J., Wagner, V. and Pálek, V.: Investigation of immunoglobulin (IgG, IgA, IgM) levels in the blood serum of uranium miners after higher and lower exposure to ionizing radiation. Strahlentherapie 149:212–218, 1975.

34. Hoover, R. and Fraumeni, J. F., Jr.: Unpublished data.

35. Roeckel, I. E.: Pathologic alterations in the lung following use of immunosuppressant agents. Ann. Clin. Lab. Sci. 3:212–218, 1973.

36. Bohan, A. and Peter, J. B.: Polymyositis and dermatomyositis. N. Engl. J. Med. 292: 344–347, 403–407, 1975.

37. Brincker, H. and Wilbek, E.: The incidence of malignant tumours in patients with respiratory sarcoidosis. Br. J. Cancer 29:247–251, 1974.

38. Brincker, H.: Personal communication.

39. Godeau, P., de Saint-Maur, P., Herreman, G. et al: Carcinome bronchiolo-alvéolaire et sclérodermie. Rapport d'une observation et revue de la littérature. Sem. Hôp. Paris 50: 1161–1168, 1974.

40. Kitagawa, M.: Autopsy study of lung cancer with special reference to scar cancer. Acta Pathol. Jap. 15:199–222, 1965.

41. McClung, J.P.: Previous pulmonary infection in lung cancer: A review. J. Chronic Dis. 20:65–78, 1967.

42. Bates, D. V.: The fate of the chronic bronchitic: A report of the ten year follow-up in the Canadian Department of Veteran's Affairs coordinated study of chronic bronchitis. Am. Rev. Respir. Dis. 108:1043–1065, 1973.

43. Baumann, H. R. and Räber, J.: Über die beziehungen zwischen Lungentuberkulose und Lungenkarzinom. Schweiz. Med. Wochenschr. 104:1774–1777, 1974.

44. Emerit, I., Levy, A. and Housset, E.: Sclérodermie généralisée et cassures chromosomiques: Mise en évidence d'un "facteur cassant" dans le sérum des malades. Ann. Génét. (Paris) 16:135–138, 1973.

45. Tolchin, S. F., Winkelstein, A., Rodnan, G. P. et al: Chromosome abnormalities from cyclophosphamide therapy in rheumatoid arthritis and progressive systemic sclerosis (scleroderma). Arthritis Rheum. 17:375–382, 1974.

46. Petitjean, R., Burghard, G., Stampfler, G. and Fievez, M.: Une nouvelle observation d'association sclérodermie et cancer alvéolaire du poumon. J. Fr. Méd. Chir. Thorac. 22:43–52, 1968.

47. Driessen, A. P. P. M. and Scherpenisse, L. A.: Familiar voorkomende diffuse interstitiële longfibrose gecompliceerd door alveolaire-cellencarcinoom. Ned Tijdschr. Geneeskd. 114:2041–2045, 1970.

48. Swaye, P., Van Ordstrand, H. S., McCormack, L. J. and Wolpaw, S. E.: Familial Hamman-Rich syndrome. Report of eight cases. Dis. Chest 55:7–12, 1969.

49. McKusick, V. A. and Fisher, A. M.: Congenital cystic disease of the lung with progressive pulmonary fibrosis and carcinomatosis. Ann. Intern. Med. 48:774–790, 1958.

50. Koch, B.: Familial fibrocystic pulmonary dysplasia: Observations in one family. Can. Med. Assoc. J. 92:801–808, 1965.

51. Vinken, P. J. and Bruyn, G. W., (eds.): The phakomatoses. In "Handbook of Clinical Neurology." New York: American Elsevier Publishing Co., Inc., 1972, vol. 14.

52. Lipton, R. A., Greenwald, R. A. and Seriff, N. S.: Pneumothorax and bilateral honeycombed lung in Marfan syndrome. Report of a case and review of the pulmonary abnormalities in this disorder. Am. Rev. Respir. Dis. 104:924–928, 1971.

53. Sosman, M. C., Dodd, G. D., Jones, W. D. and Pillmore, G. U.: The familial occurrence of pulmonary alveolar microlithiasis. Am. J. Roentgenol. Radium. Ther. Nucl. Med. 77:947–1012, 1957.

54. Wu, J. P., Gilbert, E. F. and Pellett, J. R.: Pulmonary liposarcoma in a child with adrenogenital syndrome. Am. J. Clin. Pathol. 62:791–796, 1974.

55. Tumulty, P. A.: "The Effective Clinician." Philadelphia: W. B. Saunders Company, 1973, p. 61.

56. Kloepfer, H. W., Krafchuk, J., Derbes, V. and Burks, J.: Hereditary multiple leiomyoma of the skin. Am. J. Hum. Genet. 10:48–52, 1958.

57. Freiman, D. G. and Castleman, B.: Fluctuating pulmonary shadows for twenty-two years. N. Engl. J. Med. 268:550–557, 1963.

58. Baruah, B. D. and Chari, M. V.: Kartagener's syndrome with bronchogenic carcinoma. J. Indian Med. Assoc. 21:438–439, 1952.

59. Berglund, S.: Erythrocytosis associated with haemoglobin Malmö, accompanied by pulmonary changes, occurring in the same family. Scand. J. Haematol. 9:355–369, 1972.

60. Fairbanks, V. F., Maldonado, J. E., Charache, S. and Boyer, S. H.: Familial erythrocytosis due to electrophoretically undetectable hemoglobin with impaired oxygen dissociation (hemoglobin Malmö, $\alpha_2 \beta_2^{\,97gln}$). Mayo Clin. Proc. 46:721–727, 1971.

61. Editorial: Aryl hydrocarbon hydroxylase inducibility and lung cancer. Lancet 1: 910–912, 1974.

62. Reid, W. D., Ilett, K. F., Glick, J. M. and Krishna, G.: Metabolism and binding of aromatic hydrocarbons in the lung. Am. Rev. Respir. Dis. 107:539–551, 1973.

63. Bast, R. C., Jr., Whitlock, J. P., Jr., Miller, H. et al: Aryl hydrocarbon (benzo(a)pyrene) hydroxylase in human peripheral blood monocytes. Nature 250:664–665, 1974.

64. Cantrell, E. T., Warr, G. A., Busbee, D. L. and Martin, R. R.: Induction of aryl hydrocarbon hydroxylase in human pulmonary alveolar macrophages by cigarette smoking. J. Clin. Invest. 52:1881–1884, 1973.

65. Nebert, D. W.: Genetic and environmental factors influencing drug metabolism. In Dancis, J. and Hwang, J. C. (eds.): "Perinatal Pharmacology: Problems and Priorities." New York: Raven Press, 1974.

66. Kellermann, G., Kellermann, M. L. and Shaw, C. R.: Genetic variation of aryl hydrocarbon hydroxylase in human lymphocytes. Am. J. Hum. Genet. 25:327–331, 1973.

67. Kellermann, G., Shaw, C. R. and Kellermann, M. L.: Aryl hydrocarbon hydroxylase inducibility and bronchogenic carcinoma. N. Engl. J. Med. 289:934–937, 1973.

68. Heiniger, H.-J., Taylor, B. A., Hards, E. J. and Meier, H.: Heritability of the phytohemagglutinin responsiveness of lymphocytes and its relationship to leukemogenesis. Cancer Res. 35:825–831, 1975.

69. Orell, S. R. and Mazodier, P.: Pathological findings in alpha$_1$-antitrypsin deficiency. In Mittman, C. (ed.): "Pulmonary Emphysema and Proteolysis." New York: Academic Press, Inc., 1972, pp. 69–89.

70. Anderson, A. E., Jr. and Foraker, A. G.: Comparative incidence of bronchogenic carcinoma in subjects with centrilobular and panlobular emphysema. Cancer 33:1017–1020, 1974.

71. Harris, C. C., Primack, A. and Cohen, M. H.: Elevated alpha-antitrypsin serum levels in lung cancer patients. Cancer 34:280–281, 1974.

72. Terasaki, P. I. and Mickey, M. R.: HL-A haplotypes of 32 diseases. Transplant. Rev. 22:105–119, 1975.

73. Ashley, D. J. B.: Blood groups and lung cancer. J. Med. Genet. 6:183–186, 1969.

74. Atkin, N. B.: Chromosomes in human malignant tumors: A review and assessment. In German, J. (ed.): "Chromosomes and Cancer." New York: John Wiley & Sons, 1974, pp. 375–422.

75. Makerjee, D., Trujillo, J. M., Cork, A. and Bowen, J. M.: Genetic susceptibility of human cells to transformation by oncogenic viruses. In de Grouchy, J. (ed.): "Human Genetics," ICS No. 233. Amsterdam: Excerpta Medica, 1971, p. 128.

76. Little, C. C. and Gorer, P. A.: The genetics of cancer in mice. In Grüneberg, H.: "The Genetics of the Mouse." Cambridge: University Press, 1943, pp. 311–397.

77. Heston, W. E.: Genetics: Animal tours. In Becker, F. F. (ed.): "Cancer, A Comprehensive Treatise: Etiology: Chemical and Physical Carcinogenesis." New York: Plenum Press, 1975, vol. 1, pp. 33–57.

78. Heston, W. E.: Genetics of cancer. J. Hered. 65:262–272, 1974.

79. Nomura, T.: An analysis of the changing urethan response of the developing mouse embryo in relation to mortality, malformation, and neoplasm. Cancer Res. 34:2217–2231, 1974.

80. Nomura, T.: Transmission of tumors and malformations to the next generation of mice subsequent to urethan treatment. Cancer Res. 35:264–266, 1975.

81. Nielson, S. W.: Comparative pathology of pulmonary diseases. In Liebon, A. A. and Smith, D. E. (eds.): "The Lung." Baltimore: The Williams & Wilkins Co., 1968, pp. 226–244.

82. Snyder, R. L. and Ratcliffe, H. L.: Primary lung cancers in birds and mammals of the Philadelphia zoo. Cancer Res. 26:514–518, 1966.

83. Priester, W. A. and Mantel, N.: Occurrence of tumors in domestic animals. Data from 12 United States and Canadian colleges of veterinary medicine. J. Natl. Cancer Inst. 47:1333–1344, 1971.

84. Mulvihill, J. J. and Priester, W. A.: Unpublished data.

85. Perk, K., Michalides, R., Spiegelman, S. and Schlom, J.: Biochemical and morphologic evidence for the presence of an RNA tumor virus in pulmonary carcinoma of sheep (Jaagsiekte). J. Natl. Cancer Inst. 53:131–135, 1974.

86. McKusick, V. A.: On lumpers and splitters, or the nosology of genetic disease. In Bergsma, D. (ed.): Part I, "Special Lectures," Birth Defects: Orig. Art. Ser., vol. V., no. 1. White Plains: The National Foundation–March of Dimes, 1969, pp. 23–32.

87. Pearse, A. G. E. and Polak, J. M.: Endocrine tumours of neural crest origin: Neurolo-phomas, apudomas and the apud concept. Med. Biol. 52:3–18, 1974.
88. Bolande, R. P.: The neurocristopathies. A unifying concept of disease arising in neural crest maldevelopment. Hum. Pathol. 5:409–428, 1974.
89. Weichert, R. F., III: The neural ectodermal origin of the peptide-secreting endocrine glands. A unifying concept for the etiology of multiple endocrine adenomatosis and the inappropriate secretion of peptide hormones by nonendocrine tumors. Am. J. Med. 49: 232–241, 1970.
90. Bensch, K. G., Corrin, B., Pariente, R. and Spencer, H.: Oat-cell carcinoma of the lung. Cancer 22:1163–1172, 1968.
91. Saccomanno, G., Archer, V. E., Auerbach, O. and Saunders, R. P.: Susceptibility and resistance to environmental carcinogens in the development of carcinoma of the lung. Hum. Pathol. 4:487–495, 1973.

Chromosomes and Cancer[*]

Kurt Hirschhorn, MD

During the past 10 years, there have been a number of reviews of chromosome studies in neoplasia.[1,2] Recently, an excellent book entitled "Chromosomes and Cancer," has been published. This book, edited by German, consists of a number of detailed contributions on the subject[3]; it begins with Boveri's first hypothesis on the relationship of chromosomes to malignancy,[4] and includes details on much of the information available through 1973. Therefore, this review will be confined principally to only some of the major recent findings, primarily those published in the last 2 years.

Some of the most convincing evidence that specific chromosomes may be involved in the process of neoplastic transformation or its repression is derived from several studies using somatic cell hybrids. Harris and his co-workers[5-7] produced hybrids by cell fusion using a mixture of normal and malignant cells. Such hybrids initially lose their malignant potential, which subsequently returns after the loss of chromosomes from the normal nonmalignant parent. Fusion of 2 malignant cell types results in a malignant cell, if there is no chromosome loss. If specific chromosomes are lost from such double malignant hybrids, the cells appear to lose their malignant potential. A related finding has been reported by Sachs et al who showed that duplication of specific chromosomes during propagation of polyoma transformed cells results in a suppression of malignancy.[8] Recently, Codish and Paul[9] have shown in the mouse that a specific translocation chromosome suppresses malignancy when present in 2 copies but not when present in only a single copy. All of these studies suggest that certain

*Supported in part by Genetics Center grant GM19443, NIH and Research grant HD02552, NIH.

Birth Defects: Original Article Series, Volume XII, Number 1, pages 113—121

tumors will have specific chromosomal alterations, either containing excess material resulting in the expression of malignancy or with a deletion resulting in the lack of suppression of malignancy.

In man, the classic study relating chromosomes and malignancy concerns the effects of radiation. This work, begun by Court Brown and his co-workers in patients who received heavy radiation for ankylosing spondylitis,[10] was reviewed in 1967 in a book which still is the best compilation of the relevant information.[11] Additional data of interest have been derived from the studies of the atomic bomb survivors.[12] While all of these studies demonstrated that both stable and unstable chromosomal aberrations result from radiation, it became clear that the peak of leukemia about 5 years after radiation, as well as the appearance of other tumors some 20 years after radiation, were associated with stable aberrations. These were primarily of the chromatid exchange type, leading to translocations that usually resulted in duplications and deficiencies. None of these studies, however, commented on the involvement of specific chromosomal regions, probably because they were all done before modern banding techniques became available.[13] More recently, however, early attempts at defining areas of chromosomes susceptible to radiation have been reported[14] and it is likely that future studies using the banding techniques will not only identify such susceptible regions, but may also result in the association of specific duplications and/or deficiencies to the later development of leukemia or cancer in individuals after exposure to radiation.

Studies with oncogenic viruses have resulted in the demonstration of in vitro neoplastic transformation of normal cultured cells, associated with chromosome damage. Recently, specific chromosome damage has been shown with adenovirus 12 which, in addition to producing some generalized chromosome breakage, appears to induce specific breaks in the long arm of chromosome 17 and, to a lesser extent, of chromosome 1.[15] An interesting related finding is the association of a gene controlling the SV-40 T antigen with chromosome 7,[16] and the persistence of this chromosome and the SV-40 genome in tumors produced in nude mice by cell hybrids between mouse macrophages and SV-40-transformed human cells.[17] A number of chemicals potentially or actually associated with carcinogenesis have also been shown to affect human chromosomes. Some of the best studies concern effects of streptonigrin[18] and mitomycin C.[19] With these 2 chemicals, centromeric and secondary constriction regions appear to be most susceptible to breakage and, in the case of mitomycin, rearrangements involving these regions are common. Other studies in rats also suggest preferential involvement of specific chromosomes in the formation of markers.[20] Apparently nonspecific breaks have also been described following injection of radioactive chemicals such as gold (^{198}Au)[21] and yttrium (^{90}Yt).[22] However, banding studies were not done and could conceivably have revealed specific areas of damage. Cyclophosphamide, currently used as an immunosuppressant drug, has also been shown to produce a marked increase in chromosome break-age in vivo[23] and, along with such cytotoxic agents as amethopterin, often used in psoriasis, should be considered as a possible carcinogen. While their use in the treatment of neoplasia is certainly warranted, their increasing utilization in non-neoplastic conditions is fraught with potential danger many years after the therapy. Known mutagens such as methylmetanesulphonate[24] also have been shown to produce chromosome breakage and rearrangements of types leading to stable aberrations. Most recently, polyvinyl chloride, associated with an increased incidence of liver cancer in chronically exposed workers,[25] has been shown in 2 separate studies to cause an increase in chromosome damage in vivo.[26,27]

Four diseases inherited in an autosomal recessive manner have been associated with an increased susceptibility to various forms of neoplasia and apparently spontaneous increases of chromosome breakage and rearrangement. These are Fanconi anemia,[28] Bloom syndrome,[29] ataxia-telangiectasia,[30] and xeroderma pigmentosum.[31] The last of these, associated primarily with skin cancer, shows an increased susceptibility to chromosome damage when cells from affected individuals are exposed to UV light, while the other 3 diseases show such increased susceptibility in various cells in vitro and in vivo. In Fanconi anemia, it is also possible to demonstrate an increased susceptibility of cultured skin fibroblasts to transformation by SV-40.[32] Recently, it has been suggested[33] that there is defective DNA repair in fibroblasts from Fanconi anemia patients, perhaps due to the deficiency of an exonuclease which normally removes a damaged strand of DNA after scission by endonuclease. Defective repair mechanisms have also been suggested for the Bloom syndrome in which the most likely defect would appear to be in one form of DNA polymerase, leading to a retarded rate of DNA chain growth.[34] The clearest demonstration of defective repair mechanisms has been in xeroderma pigmentosum.[35] While this condition in general has been thought to be due to the deficiency of at least one of the enzymes involved in excision repair of UV-induced damage to DNA,[36] a great deal of genetic heterogeneity has been demonstrated. There are, for example, 5 complementation groups, as detected by somatic cell hybridization experiments.[37] Perhaps another subgroup of xeroderma patients is defective in DNA synthesis after UV irradiation, enhanced by caffeine, but with normal levels of excision repair.[38] Other workers have suggested a decreased level of photore-activating enzyme.[39] Chromosome damage in xeroderma pigmentosum cells is also enhanced by adenovirus 12.[40] A good review of DNA repair in mammalian cells has been published recently by Strauss.[41] It is clear that x-ray and UV-irradiation have a synergistic effect on chromosome breakage in normal cells,[42] and it has been suggested that perhaps most aberrations — whether caused by radiation or by a variety of chemical agents — are the consequences of the defective operation of repair mechanisms, DNA replication, and the action of a single strand of DNAase.[43] Although no defect in repair mechanisms has yet been reported in ataxia-telangiectasia, there is a suggestion of involvement of a specific chromosome (number 14) in the markers found in patients with this syndrome.[44] It is of related interest that sporadic translocations found in a small number of cells of short-term lymphoid cultures from normal individuals apparently preferentially consist of rearrangements involving chromosomes 7 and 14.[45–47] The latter of these is associated with the premalignant disease ataxia-telangiectasia, while rearrangements involving number 7, at least in the form of a deletion, seem to be associated with some forms of leukemia.[48] It is also of interest that we have demonstrated at least partial homology of part of the long arm of a D group (13–15) chromosome and the feline C-type virus RD-114.[49] In the Bloom syndrome specific regions of chromosomes appear to be preferentially affected and participate in the relatively typical lesion observed, that of interchanges involving homologous sites in homologous chromosomes.[50] Recently, a new technique has been described by Latt[51] which can accurately define sister chromatid exchange. The technique has been simplified by Perry and Wolff.[52] Lymphocytes from patients with the Bloom syndrome exhibit a massive increase in such exchanges[53] which is not seen in Fanconi anemia or ataxia-telangiectasia, and which may be due to damage occurring during S (DNA synthesis) or during G2 in interphase cells.

The classic association between a specific chromosome abnormality and a specific neoplastic state is that of the Philadelphia chromosome with chronic myelogenous leukemia.[54] Although first believed to be a deletion of half of the long arm of chromosome 22,[55] recent studies have shown that the aberration actually is a translocation, usually between chromosome 22 and 9,[56] but occasionally involving another chromosome with number 22.[57] Additional changes may occur in the leukemic cells during blastic crises, some of which appear to be nonspecific,[58] although a not infrequent secondary change appears to be the loss of the Y chromosome in males with the disease.[59] In view of the fact that the entire marrow and its products, with the exception of the lymphoid elements, is often populated by Philadelphia chromosome positive cells, and that all of these cells have been shown to derive clonally from a single cell, as demonstrated by their sharing of the same active X in affected females heterozygous for an X-linked marker[60] it would appear that the chromosomal event occurs before the development of the disease. A similar specific abnormality, apparent deletion of the long arm of chromosome 20, although not nearly as common, has been found in some patients with myeloproliferative disorders, especially polycythemia vera and sideroblastic anemia.[61,62] Additional abnormalities in polycythemia have included an extra chromosome 8 or 9.[63] It is of great interest that Rowley[48] and others[64] have shown the involvement of an extra chromosome 8, an extra chromosome 9, and the loss of all or part of a chromosome 7, or the X, as the most common chromosomal variations in leukemia as well. Of these, an extra chromosome 8 is by far the most common. Although some additional chromosomal abnormalities have been reported in acute leukemia, the previous concept of randomness of damage appears to have been in error and, if it occurs later in the evolution of the neoplasm, may represent effects secondary to and resulting from the primary chromosomal aberration. It certainly would appear that the existence of abnormal cytogenetic findings in the bone marrow of such patients is associated with a poor prognosis.[65]

Studies of nonleukemic neoplasms are also gradually revealing specific chromosome abnormalities. These include meningiomas with a loss of number 22,[66,67] an additional terminal fluorescent band on number 14 in tumors of some patients with Burkitt lymphoma,[68] and the loss of a portion of the long arm of 13 in some cases of retinoblastoma.[69] The loss of the Y chromosome has also been reported in a fairly high percentage of solid malignant tumors.[70]

In view of the various findings just discussed, it would appear more and more likely that chromosome damage of a relatively specific nature is associated with the primary event responsible for neoplastic transformation of a cell. Certainly the preexistence of chromosome damage in the chromosome breakage syndromes, the increased susceptibility to neoplasia in the Down syndrome,[71] the detection of x-ray—induced chromosome damage long before the discovery of neoplasia, and the specificity of chromosome abnormalities associated with specific neoplasms, such as chronic myelogenous leukemia, derived from single cells, lends credence to the concept that specific chromosome imbalance may be primary events in tumorigenesis. This imbalance may be reflected either by loss of growth controlling genes, the duplication of genes acting in the opposite direction, or even specific gene loss or position effect produced by translocations. The relevant gene loci or regions may well be associated with vertically transmitted information able to code for viral genomes such as chromosome 7 for SV-40.[17] Similar conclusions are developing from work in other animals. For example, trisomy 15 has been found in spontaneous leukemia in AKR mice[72] and chromosomal localization of genes responsible for the synthesis of C-type particles after exposure to carcinogens[73] or desoxynucleoside analogs[74] has been achieved.[75] It is therefore possible, as we have suggested previously,[76] that oncogenic viruses may in fact be the products of inherited genes which are activated during neoplastic transformation by chemicals or irradiation, or even during chromosome breakage and rearrangement. These viruses therefore may not be primarily responsible for the oncogenic state but, by producing new antigens or reactivating fetal antigens on the surface of the cell, may serve to protect the organism by allowing immunologic recognition and killing of transformed cells. The partial homology between some of these viruses derived from various species including man[77,78] indicates relative evolutionary stability for such putative genes, and implies a beneficial role or selective advantage. Failure of expression of the new cellular antigenicity, inadequate cellular immunity, or even inappropriate humoral immunity producing blocking antibodies,[79] may then result in the uninhibited growth of the abnormal cell.

In summary, the new banding techniques are providing a growing body of information which relates specific chromosome aberrations to various forms of leukemia and cancer. Studies of the localization of chromosome damage induced by known possible oncogenic agents may allow correlation between such agents and the specific tumors they may cause. Additional new techniques, such as the detection of sister chromatid exchange and the accurate mapping and immunologic study of viruses associated with neoplasia, may help in understanding the mechanisms involved in the relationship between chromosomes and cancer.

REFERENCES

1. Hirschhorn, K.: Cytogenetic alterations in leukemia. In "Perspectives in Leukemia," New York: Grune and Stratton, 1968, p. 113.
2. Hirschhorn, K.: Cytogenetic and immunologic abnormalities related to leukemia. In "6th National Cancer Conference Proceedings," Philadelphia: J. B. Lippincott, 1970, p. 107.
3. German, J. (ed.): "Chromosomes and Cancer," New York: John Wiley and Sons, 1974.
4. Boveri, T.: "Zur Frage der Entstehung Maligner Tumoren," Jena: Gustav Fischer, 1914.
5. Klein, G., Bregula, U., Wiener, F. and Harris, H.: The analysis of malignancy by cell fusion. I. Hybrids between tumor cells and L cell derivatives. J. Cell Sci. 8:659, 1971.
6. Harris, H.: Cell fusion and the analysis of malignancy. Proc. R. Soc. 179:1, 1971.
7. Wiener, F., Klein, G. and Harris, H.: The analysis of malignancy by cell fusion. IV. Hybrids between tumour cells and a malignant L cell derivative. J. Cell Sci. 12:253, 1973.
8. Hitotsumachi, S., Rabinowitz, Z. and Sachs, L.: Chromosomal control of reversion in transformed cells. Nature 231:511, 1972.
9. Codish, S. D. and Paul, B.: Reversible appearance of a specific chromosome which suppresses malignancy. Nature 252:610, 1974.
10. Tough, I. M., Buckton, K. E., Baikie, A. G. and Court Brown, W. M.: X-ray-induced chromosome damage in man. Lancet 2:849, 1960.
11. Evans, H. J., Court Brown, W. M. and McLean, A. S. (eds.): "Human Radiation Cytogenetics," Amsterdam: North Holland Publishing Co., 1967.
12. Bloom, A. D.: Induced chromosomal aberrations in man. In "Advances in Human Genetics." Harris, H. and Hirschhorn, K. (eds.): New York: Plenum Press, 1972, vol. 3, pp. 99–172.
13. Hirschhorn, K.: Chromosome identification. Annu. Rev. Med. 24:67, 1973.
14. Seabright, M.: High resolution studies on the pattern of induced exchanges in the human karyotype. Chromosoma 40:333, 1973.
15. McDougall, J. K.: Adenovirus-induced chromosome aberrations in human cells. J. Gen. Virol. 12:43, 1971.
16. Croce, C. M. and Koprowski, H.: Concordant segregation of the expression of SV-40 T antigen and human chromosome 7 in mouse-human hybrid subclones. J. Exp. Med. 139:1350, 1974.

17. Croce, C. M., Aden, D. and Koprowski, H.: Somatic cell hybrids between mouse peritoneal macrophages and simian-virus-40-transformed human cells: II. Presence of human chromosome 7 carrying simian virus 40 genome in cells of tumor induced by hybrid cells. Proc. Natl. Acad. Sci. USA 72:1397, 1975.

18. Cohen, M. M.: The specific effects of streptonigrin activity on human leukocytes in culture. Cytogenetics 2:271, 1963.

19. Cohen, M. M. and Shaw, M. W.: Effects of mitomycin C on human chromosomes. J. Cell Biol. 23:386, 1964.

20. Olini, C. D. and DiPaolo, J. A.: Chromosome binding patterns of rat fibrosarcomas induced by in vitro transformation of embryo cells or in vivo injection of rats by 7, 12-dimethylbenz-(alpha) anthracene. J. Natl. Cancer Inst. 52:1627, 1974.

21. Stevenson, A. C., Bedford, J., Hill, A. G. S. and Hill, H.: Chromosome damage in patients who have had intra-articular injections of radioactive gold. Lancet 1:837, 1971.

22. de La Chapelle, A., Oka, M., Rekonen, A. and Ruotsi, A.: Chromosome damage after intra-articular injections of radioactive yttrium. Ann. Rheum. Dis. 31:508, 1972.

23. Tolchin, S. F., Winkelstein, A. Rodnan, G. P. et al: Chromosome abnormalities from cyclophosphamide therapy in rheumatoid arthritis and progressive systemic sclerosis (scleroderma). Arthritis Rheum. 17:375, 1974.

24. Brøgger, A.: Different patterns of chromosome exchange induced by methyl-metanesulphonate and mitomycin C in human cells. Hereditas 77:205, 1974.

25. Creech, J. L. and Johnson, M. N.: Angiosarcoma of liver in the manufacture of vinyl chloride. J. Occup. Med. 16:150, 1974.

26. Ducatman, A., Hirschhorn, K. and Selikoff, I. J.: Vinyl chloride exposure in human chromosome aberrations. Mutat. Res. 31:163, 1975.

27. Funes-Cravioto, F., Lambert, B., Lindsten, J. et al: Chromsome aberrations in workers exposed to vinyl chloride. Lancet 1:349, 1975.

28. Swift, M. and Hirschhorn, K.: Fanconi's anemia. Ann. Intern. Med. 65:496, 1966.

29. Sawitsky, A., Bloom, D. and German, J.: Chromosomal breakage and acute leukemia in congenital telangiectatic erythema and stunted growth. Ann. Intern. Med. 65:487, 1966.

30. Hecht, F., Koler, R. D., Rigas, D. A. et al: Leukaemia and lymphocytes in ataxia telangiectasia. Lancet 2:1193, 1966.

31. German, J.: Genes which increase chromosomal instability in somatic cells and predispose to cancer. Prog. Med. Genet. 8:61, 1972.

32. Todaro, G. J., Green, H. and Swift, M. R.: Susceptibility of human diploid fibroblast strains to transformation by SV-40 virus. Science 153:1252, 1966.

33. Poon, P. K., O'Brien, R. L. and Parker, J. W.: Defective DNA repair in Fanconi's anaemia. Nature 250:223, 1974.

34. Hand, R. and German, J.: A retarded rate of DNA chain growth in Bloom's syndrome. Proc. Natl. Acad. Sci. USA 72:758, 1975.

35. Cleaver, J. E.: Defective repair replication of DNA in xeroderma pigmentosum. Nature 218:652, 1968.

36. Setlow, R. B., Regan, J. D., German, J. and Carrier, W. L.: Evidence that xeroderma pigmentosum cells do not perform the first step in the repair of ultraviolet damage to their DNA. Proc. Natl. Acad. Sci. USA 64:1035, 1969.

37. Kraemer, K. H., Coon, H. G., Petinga, R. A. et al: Genetic heterogeneity in xeroderma pigmentosum: Complementation groups and their relationship to DNA repair rates. Proc. Natl. Acad. Sci. USA 72:59, 1975.

38. Lehmann, A. R., Kirk-Bell, S., Arlett, C. F. et al: Xeroderma pigmentosum cells with

normal levels of excision repair have a defect in DNA synthesis after UV-irradiation. Proc. Natl. Acad. Sci. USA 72:219, 1975.

39. Sutherland, B. M., Rice, M. and Wagner, E. K.: Xeroderma pigmentosum cells contain low levels of photoreactivating enzyme. Proc. Natl. Acad. Sci. USA 72:103, 1975.

40. Stich, H. F., Stich, W. and Lam, P.: Susceptibility of xeroderma pigmentosum cells to chromosome breakage by adenovirus type 12. Nature 250:599, 1974.

41. Strauss, B. S.: Repair of DNA in mammalian cells. Life Sci. 15:1685, 1974.

42. Holmberg, M. and Jonasson, J.: Synergistic effect of x-ray and UV-irradiation on the frequency of chromosome breakage in human lymphocytes. Mutat. Res. 23:213, 1974.

43. Bender, M. A., Griggs, H. G. and Bedford, J. S.: Mechanisms of chromosomal aberration production. III. Chemicals and ionizing radiation. Mutat. Res. 23:197, 1974.

44. Harnden, D. G.: Ataxia telangiectasia syndrome: Cytogenetic and cancer aspects. In "Chromosomes and Cancer," op. cit. p. 619.

45. Welch, J. P. and Lee, C. L. Y.: Non-random occurrence of 7–14 translocations in human lymphocyte cultures. Nature 255:241, 1975.

46. Beatty-DeSana, J. W., Hoggard, M. J. and Cooledge, J. W.: Non-random occurrence of 7–14 translocations in human lymphocyte cultures. Nature 255:242, 1975.

47. Hecht, F. and McCaw, B. K.: Non-random occurrence of 7–14 translocations in human lymphocyte cultures. Nature 255:243, 1975.

48. Rowley, J. D.: Nonrandom chromosomal abnormalities in hematologic disorders of man. Proc. Natl. Acad. Sci. USA 72:152, 1975.

49. Price, P. M., Hirschhorn, K., Gabelman, N. and Waxman, S.: In situ hybridization of RD114-virus RNA with human metaphase chromosomes. Proc. Natl. Acad. Sci. USA 70:11, 1973.

50. German, J., Crippa, L. P. and Bloom, D.: Bloom's syndrome. III. Analysis of the chromosome aberration characteristic of this disorder. Chromosoma 48:361, 1974.

51. Latt, S. A.: Microfluorometric detection of deoxyribonucleic acid replication in human metaphase chromosomes. Proc. Natl. Acad. Sci. USA 70:3395, 1973.

52. Perry, P. and Wolff, S.: A new Giemsa method for the differential staining of sister chromatids. Nature (In press.)

53. Chaganti, R. S. K., Schonberg, S. and German, J.: A manifold increase in sister chromatid exchanges in Bloom's syndrome lymphocytes. Proc. Natl. Acad. Sci. USA 71:4508, 1974.

54. Nowell, P. C. and Hungerford, D. A.: A minute chromosome in human CML. Science 132:1497, 1960.

55. Caspersson, T., Gahrton, G., Lindsten, J. and Zech, L.: Identification of the Philadelphia chromosome as no. 22 by quinacrine mustard fluorescence analysis. Exp. Cell Res. 63:238, 1970.

56. Rowley, J. D.: A new consistent chromosomal abnormality in chronic myelogenous leukemia identified by quinacrine fluorescence and Giemsa staining. Nature 243:290, 1973.

57. Gahrton, G., Zech, L. and Lindsten, J.: A new variant translocation ($19q^+$, $22q^-$) in chronic myelocytic leukemia. Exp. Cell Res. 86:214, 1974.

58. Fitzgerald, P. H.: A complex pattern of chromosome abnormalities in the acute phase of CML. J. Med. Genet. 3:258, 1966.

59. Lawler, S. D., Loss, D. S. and Wiltshaw, E.: Philadelphia-chromosome positive bone-marrow cells showing loss of the Y in males with chronic myeloid leukaemia. Br. J. Haematol. 27:247, 1974.

60. Fialkow, P. J., Gartler, S. M. and Yoshida, A.: Clonal origin of CML in man. Proc. Natl. Acad. Sci. USA 58:1468, 1967.

61. Kay, H. E. M., Lawler, S. D. and Millard, R. E.: The chromosomes in polycythemia vera. Br. J. Haematol. 12:507, 1966.
62. Cohen, M. D., Ariel, I. and Dagan, J.: Chromosome deletion (46,XY, 20q⁻) in sideroblastic anemia. Isr. J. Med. Sci. 10:1393, 1974.
63. Hsu, L. Y. F., Alter, A. V. and Hirschhorn, K.: Trisomy 8 in bone marrow cells of patients with polycythemia vera and myelogenous leukemia. Clin. Genet. 6:258, 1974.
64. Jonasson, J., Gahrton, G., Lindsten, J. et al: Trisomy 8 in acute myeloblastic leukemia and sideroachrestic anemia. Blood 43:557, 1974.
65. Sakurai, M. and Sandberg, A. A.: Chromosomes and causation of human cancer and leukemia. IX. Prognostic and therapeutic value of chromosomal findings in acute myeloblastic leukemia. Cancer 33:1548, 1974.
66. Zankl, H. and Zang, K. D.: Cytological and cytogenetical studies on brain tumors. IV. Identification of the missing G chromosome in human meningiomas as No. 22 by fluorescence technique. Humangenetik 14:167, 1972.
67. Mark, J., Levan, G. and Mitelman, F.: Identification by fluorescence of the G chromosome lost in human meningiomas. Hereditas 71:163, 1972.
68. Manalov, G. and Manalova, Y.: Marker band in one chromosome 14 from Burkitt's lymphoma. Nature 237:33, 1972.
69. Wilson, M. G., Towner, J. W. and Fujimoto, A.: Retinoblastoma and D-chromosome deletions. Am. J. Hum. Genet. 25:57, 1973.
70. Sellyei, M. and Vass, L.: Sex-chromosome loss in human tumours. Lancet 1:1041, 1975.
71. Holland, S. N., Doll, R. and Carter, C. O.: The mortality from leukaemia and other causes among patients with Down's syndrome and among their parents. Br. J. Cancer 16:177, 1962.
72. Dofuku, R., Biedler, J. L., Spengler, B. A. and Old, L. J.: Trisomy of chromosome 15 in spontaneous leukemia of AKR mice. Proc. Natl. Acad. Sci. USA 72:1515, 1975.
73. Rowe, W. P., Lowy, D. R., Teich, N. and Hartley, J. W.: Some implications of the activation of murine leukemia virus by halogenated pyrimidines. Proc. Natl. Acad. Sci. USA 69:1033, 1972.
74. Lieber, M. M., Benveniste, R. E., Livingston, D. M. and Todaro, G. I.: Mammalian cells in culture frequently release type C viruses. Science 182:56, 1973.
75. Rowe, W. P., Hartley, J. W. and Bremner, T.: Genetic mapping of a murine leukemia virus-inducing locus of AKR mice. Science 178:860, 1972.
76. Hirschhorn, K., Price, P. M., Gabelman, N. and Waxman, S.: Evolutionary significance of persistence of latent oncogenic virus information in vertebrates. Lancet 1:1158, 1973.
77. Axel, R., Schlom, J. and Spiegelman, S.: Presence in human breast cancer of RNA homologous to mouse mammary tumor virus RNA. Nature 235:32, 1972.
78. Benveniste, R. E. and Todaro, G. J.: Evolution of C-type viral genes: Inheritance of exogenously acquired viral genes. Nature 252:456, 1974.
79. Hellstrom, K. E. and Hellstrom, I.: Immunological enhancement as studied by cell culture techniques. Annu. Rev. Microbiol. 24:373, 1970.

Human Tumors Studied with Genetic Markers[*]

Philip J. Fialkow, MD

Because direct studies of tumor formation cannot be done in man, most investigations provide only indirect evidence about causative factors. One such indirect approach involves the use of genetic markers to determine the number of cells from which tumors arise, thereby providing important clues to their mode of origin. For example, a neoplasm that results from a rare event like "spontaneous" somatic mutation will arise in a single cell. On the other hand, multicellular origin would be anticipated if a growth arises primarily as a result of cell-to-cell spread of an oncogenic virus. This problem can be investigated by studying tumors in subjects with at least 2 genetically marked populations of cells, ie in those with cellular mosaicism. To illustrate this point, assume that a patient has 2 types of cells in equal frequency, one identifiable by marker A and the other by marker B. Tumors of unicellular (clonal) origin contain only one type of cell, A or B, whereas both types would be likely in neoplasms arising in many cells.

Immunoglobulin markers were first employed for this purpose,[1] but they are useful only in neoplasms within the immune system. More generally applicable cell-marker systems are dependent upon X-chromosome inactivation mosaicism. They can be used to investigate all tumors that arise in subjects with appropriate X-linked markers. Especially useful for this purpose is the cellular mosaicism of females heterozygous for the X-linked glucose-6-phosphate dehydrogenase (G-6-PD). Females who carry a gene for the usual type of G-6-PD (Gd^B) on one X chromosome and the common variant Gd^A gene on the other, have 2 cell populations, one producing G-6-PD type A, and the other, G-6-PD type B. The

*Supported by USPHS Research Grants GM 15253 and CA 16448 from the National Institutes of Health.

Birth Defects: Original Article Series, Volume XII, Number 1, pages 123–132

2 isoenzymes have different electrophoretic mobility and are easily distinguishable. Tumors with clonal origin exhibit only one type of enzyme (A or B), whereas those arising from multiple cells might have both A and B enzymes. The electrophoretic variants are prevalent only in blacks. Thus, this approach is best applied to the study of tumors in black females; in many areas of the world 35–45% of these women are G-6-PD heterozygotes. This system, first utilized to demonstrate clonal origin of uterine leiomyomas,[2] has been employed to study many neoplasms. In this communication, 2 diseases studied in the author's laboratory, chronic myelocytic leukemia and Burkitt lymphoma, are discussed in detail. More extensive reviews appear elsewhere.[3,4]

CHRONIC MYELOCYTIC LEUKEMIA (CML)

Bone-marrow cells from the majority of CML patients have a specific and characteristic translocation involving chromosome 22 and generally chromosome 9.[5] This Philadelphia (Ph[1]) chromosome rearrangement, which may be found even before the onset of overt leukemia,[6] is undoubtedly important in the pathogenesis of the disease. However, the primary causes of CML (presumably, the factors which induce the Ph[1] abnormality) are unknown. Important clues to the mode of origin can be provided through determination of the number of cells from which CML arises. In most cases 90–100% of dividing marrow cells are Ph[1]-positive, but this fact does not necessarily indicate clonal origin of the disease; it is conceivable that Ph[1] arises independently in many cells.

Six G-6-PD heterozygotes with Ph[1]-positive CML have been studied.[7–9] As expected, both B and A enzymes were found in cultured skin fibroblasts, but in each case only a single enzyme type was observed in the leukemic granulocytes (3 patients had type A and 3 patients had type B). These findings in CML cells are in marked contrast to those in blood cells from G-6-PD heterozygotes without leukemia, which almost invariably exhibit both B and A enzymes.[10] Therefore, the single enzyme phenotypes in CML are related to the disease and most probably reflect a clonal origin. However, since there are other conceivable explanations for single enzyme phenotypes, it was important to confirm the G-6-PD findings with other systems. This has been done by studies with another isoenzyme[11,12] and with chromosomal markers.[13–17] Thus, clonal origin of CML seems firmly established, but obviously this conclusion applies only to the stage in which the disease is clinically apparent. Conceivably, at an earlier phase a number of cells might be affected, but by the time leukemia can be diagnosed, one clone has evolved.

In which type of cell does CML arise? Is it a cell already committed to become a granulocyte or is it a more primordial stem cell? Erythrocytes as well as granulocytes of the 3 tested Gd^B/Gd^A heterozygotes contained only enzyme type A.[7] In contrast, both B and A enzymes are found in erythrocytes of non-leukemic Gd^B/Gd^A heterozygotes.[10] Thus, the leukemia clone arise in a stem cell common to the erythrocyte and granulocyte, but not to the skin fibroblast. This conclusion is supported by the demonstration of the Ph^1 rearrangement in erythrocyte precursors.[18, 19] In as yet unpublished studies, we have observed single enzyme phenotypes in platelets and cultured monocytes from a G-6-PD heterozygote with CML. G-6-PD typing of lymphocytes has not been reported, but blood lymphocytes stimulated to divide in vitro by phytohemagglutinin (PHA) apparently are Ph^1-negative. The latter cells are presumably T lymphocytes and the absence of Ph^1 in them cannot be expanded into a general interpretation regarding all classes of lymphocytes. For example, those lymphocytes which are non-PHA responsive (eg B lymphocytes) may be descendants of the CML stem cell. Furthermore, PHA-responsive cells are long-lived and, therefore, may have antedated the occurrence of CML.

Another question and one which is relevant to therapy is: Are there any normal stem cells in CML? The facts that the proportion of Ph^1-positive dividing marrow cells does not decline in remission and that the single-enzyme G-6-PD phenotypes persist indicate that the marrow is not repopulated with normal stem cells. Nonetheless, these observations do not exclude the presence of a very small population of normal stem cells, which, if it contributed less than 5% of the dividing marrow cells or 5–10% of the total enzyme activity, might not be detected. That there may be such cells is suggested by the observations of a few Ph^1-negative colonies in cultured stem cells from some patients with CML[20] and by occasional reports of CML patients with unusual sensitivity to chemotherapy, who after recovery from profound marrow depression develop a Ph^1-negative population.[21]

The Ph^1-chromosome rearrangement may well be the immediate cause of CML, but the primary causes that presumably induce Ph^1 remain largely unknown. Among possible etiologic factors are rare "spontaneous" or radiation-induced genetic accidents, viruses and physiologic defects in marrow homeostasis. The mutation hypothesis predicts single cell origin and the G-6-PD data are in accord with this suggestion. The defective homeostasis hypothesis implies that the basic abnormality is not intrinsic to the marrow cells themselves, but is found in the mechanisms which regulate marrow proliferation and differentiation. Insofar as this hypothesis predicts multicellular origin, the genetic marker data make it unlikely to be correct. Viral- or radiation-induced origin could be from one or many cells. For example, the oncogenic change induced by a virus could be rare, giving rise to a single clone; alternatively, the putative oncogenic virus might have specificity for the involved regions on chromosomes 22 and 9, in which case Ph^1 could be induced in multiple cells. The latter mechanism is rendered very unlikely by the finding that CML has a clonal origin. This fact also virtually excludes any hypothesis of pathogenesis

based on continuous cell recruitment (ie the ability of a cell that has undergone leukemic transformation to induce continuously other cells to become
a part of the neoplasm, possibly by transfer of an infectious agent).

Since CML is often associated with prolonged survival unless myelofibrosis
or acute blastic transformation occurs, it can be regarded as a preleukemic
condition. The factors that govern progression to malignant leukemia are
unknown. Genetic marker studies indicate that blastic transformation occurs
in preexisting CML cells and one possibility is that a single CML cell undergoes
transformation and gives rise to the acute leukemia-like clone. Alternatively,
the blasts originate from multiple CML cells. G-6-PD studies do not permit
distinction between these 2 possibilities, since by the time blastic transformation occurs, all or most of the hematopoietic cells are already derived from a
single clone. However, chromosomal markers indicate that a CML subclone
evolves to blastic transformation.[22–24]

Many other neoplasms have been studied with the G-6-PD system and the
data suggest that most of them have clonal origin.[3,4] What types of tumor might
one expect to have multicellular origin? One possibility is a neoplasm that de-
velops in a subject with an innate predisposition to tumorigenesis such as might
be seen in a patient with a genetic disease strongly associated with tumor
formation.

HEREDITARY NEUROFIBROMATOSIS

Neurofibromas from patients with the dominantly inherited syndrome of multiple neurofibromatosis (von Recklinghausen disease) have double enzyme phenotypes indicating multicellular origin.[25] One alternate possibility to explain the
double enzyme phenotypes, that the neurofibromas contain both B and A enzymes because they are "contaminated" with nonneoplastic cells such as inflammatory cells, stroma, etc, has been excluded by careful histologic studies.
The suggestion that both G-6-PD genes are active in individual neurofibroma
cells can be discounted because no electrophoretic band intermediate in migration between A and B was observed. G-6-PD is a dimer and when both genes are
active in a single cell a hybrid molecule of A and B subunits is formed.

The mosaic composition of a hereditary neurofibroma is practically identical
to that of the overlying normal skin; therefore, it is probable that the neoplasm
originates from hundreds or even thousands of cells. The initial tumorigenic
step is germinal mutation, but since the neurofibroma starts from so many cells,
subsequent steps in tumor development are not rare mutation-like events.
Rather, a relatively large number of cells may be simultaneously affected by the
tumorigenic process as might be seen with neoplasms induced by hormonal
changes. Increased levels of nerve growth factor have been described in patients
with hereditary neurofibromatosis.[26] Alternatively, origin of a tumor from

hundreds of cells could be seen if the oncogenic mechanism initially altered only a single cell and this alteration subsequently influenced the pattern of growth in neighboring cells.

Double enzyme phenotypes are also a feature of dominantly inherited multiple trichoepithelioma.[27] However, since this neoplasm is heterogeneous with respect to cell composition (ie fibroblasts and epithelium), the significance of the G-6-PD phenotypes is open to question.

What other circumstances might underlie tumors with multiple cell origin? In addition to innate susceptibility, the nature of the external etiologic agent may be a major factor in determining the number of cells affected. For example, multicellular origin will occur when tumors are caused by cell-to-cell spread and transformation by oncogenic viruses. Similarly, this might be detected for neoplasms strongly influenced by hormones.

WARTS

The only neoplasms in man with proven viral cause are warts. We elected to study "venereal" warts (condyloma acuminata), growths which are caused by a papova virus and occur at mucocutaneous junctions, such as the vulva. Each lesion consists of cauliflower-like clumps of small individual verrucous subunits. Double enzyme phenotypes were found in each of 4 warts from 2 G-6-PD heterozygotes.[28] Furthermore, epithelial remnants from even the smallest verrucal subunits occasionally had double enzyme phenotypes. Thus, the hypothesis that at least some growths caused by a virus have multicellular origin is confirmed.

In contrast to the findings in condyloma acuminata, single enzyme phenotypes were reported in each of 6 common warts (verrucca vulgaris) from as many patients.[29] These findings are compatible with clonal origin. An alternative explanation is that the common wart arises from several cells but that in each of the 6 common warts studied all the transformed cells happened to have the same G-6-PD phenotype. If this interpretation were correct, further study of common warts should reveal some with double enzyme phenotypes.

BURKITT LYMPHOMA

A malignant disease for which there is much circumstantial evidence of a viral cause in man is Burkitt lymphoma. The putative agent is Epstein-Barr virus (EBV), a ubiquitous DNA herpesvirus. Data implicating this virus are the elevated titers of EBV-related antibodies in African children with Burkitt lymphoma[30–32] and the presence of EBV genomes in Burkitt tumor cells, [33] which also have a very characteristic, virally determined nuclear antigen.[34] EBV genomes have not been detected in the cells of any other lymphoma. Although these data are suggestive, there is no direct evidence that EBV is a cause of Burkitt lymphoma. In fact, it has been suggested that the virus is merely a passenger in the lymphoblastoid cells. A strong argument against the passenger hypothesis can be made on the basis of findings in the rare cases of "Burkitt lymphoma" that occur in the United States and other nonendemic areas. Despite the facts that EBV is ubiquitous and these cases are histologically and clinically indistinguishable from African Burkitt lymphoma, the tumor cells lack EBV genomes,[35,36] suggesting a fundamental difference between African and American Burkitt lymphoma.

Single enzyme phenotypes have been found in 45 of 46 Burkitt tumors obtained from 29 G-6-PD heterozygotes ascertained at the Kenyatta National Hospital in Nairobi.[37-39] In contrast, both enzyme types were found in the patient's normal tissues including blood lymphocytes, lymph nodes, ovaries, etc. Although other explanations cannot be overlooked, it seems most likely that these observations reflect clonal origin of the great majority of Burkitt tumors. The one neoplasm with a double enzyme phenotype could have arisen from 2 or more clones. Alternatively, the portions of this tumor subjected to starch-gel electrophoresis may have been contaminated by nontumor cells.

On initial presentation, patients with Burkitt lymphoma usually have tumors at multiple anatomic sites. Consequently, one may ask: Does the entire disease have clonal origin, ie does it begin in one site and then spread to other parts of the body, or does each of the tumors arise independently of the others? If each tumor arises independently, one expects to find some neoplasms of type B and others of type A in the same patient. On the other hand, if Burkitt lymphoma begins in a single cell at one site and then spreads to other parts of the body, all tumors in the same patient should have the same single enzyme type. Two tumors were studied from each of 11 patients and in all cases the 2 tumors were concordant.[38] The probability that this degree of concordance would occur by chance alone is less than 1%. Thus, it seems likely that Burkitt lymphoma is a clonal disease beginning in one site and then spreading to other parts of the body.

Single cell origin of the putative viral malignancy has important pathogenetic implications; therefore, it was of considerable importance to confirm the G-6-PD findings with another marker system. Since Burkitt cells frequently synthesize immunoglobulin which may be found on their surfaces, cell-surface immunoglobulin mosaicism can be utilized for this purpose. Data derived from study of over 100 Burkitt tumors strongly support the conclusions reached with the G-6-PD system.[38]

Does the probable unicellular origin of Burkitt lymphoma argue against the disease's putative viral etiology? Although viruses infect many cells, clonal origin of a neoplasm does not exclude a viral cause. There are at least 4 circumstances in which a virally induced neoplasm might have single cell origin: 1) If the oncogenic change induced by the virus were relatively rare, such as a somatic gene or chromosome mutation-like event. A specific chromosome alteration in Burkitt lymphoma has been described.[40] 2) If the virus were a necessary but not a sufficient etiologic factor and one of the other tumorigenic co-factors affected only a single cell. 3) If the development of the tumor were dependent upon the step-wise accumulation of several changes, such that accumulation of the required number and sequence in a single cell would be a rare event; and 4) If many cells were altered by the virus, but once a malignant clone emerged, the growth of other clones was inhibited. In any event, the single cell origin of the *malignant* putative viral disease, Burkitt lymphoma, contrasts with the multicellular origin of the *benign* viral growth, "venereal" wart. This difference suggests that virus-infected cells give rise to a malignant clone only if one or more additional events occurs.

Most patients with Burkitt lymphoma have therapeutically induced "complete" remissions, but tumors reappear within a year in about 60% of cases.[41,42] Are these true recurrences of old disease (ie reemergence of the original tumor cell line), or are they newly induced malignant clones? The first studied G-6-PD heterozygote with a relatively late remission at an anatomically distant site, was a 6-year-old girl who on initial presentation had ovarian and parotid tumors.[43] Normal tissues were typed as B/A for G-6-PD. Only the ovarian tumor was tested; it was typed as B. The patient had a chemotherapeutically induced "complete" remission followed by exacerbation of disease in the left parotid gland (a site previously affected by tumor). Like the original ovarian neoplasm, the recurrent parotid tumor was typed as B. A second remission was induced, but this was followed by exacerbation in the orbit, a previously uninvolved anatomic site. In contrast to the initial tumors, the orbit relapse was typed as A. Thus, in this patient, exacerbation of disease in a previously uninvolved site did not result from reemergence of the malignant cell line originally detected. In 2 of 8 other patients with relapses occurring after 5 months, discordant immunoglobulin phenotypes were found in the recurrent tumors. These findings contrast with those of 27 early (under 3 months) recurrent tumors which were uniformly concordant with the phenotypes found in the initial tumors.[38] Thus, it is concluded that early relapses are reemergences of the original malignant clones, but some "late" recurrences may be the result of newly induced malignant clones.

Ziegler and associates[42] made a similar suggestion on the basis of clinical observations. They noted that early relapses appear at previously involved anatomic sites, whereas late regrowths often occur in previously uninvolved organs. Furthermore, the proportion of late relapses which have favorable therapeutic responses is similar to what is found in primary tumors, whereas early relapses almost always have poor responses. Therefore, it was suggested that most early relapses are due to reemergences of the original malignant clones, while some late recurrences may be due to emergence of new malignant cell lines.

ACUTE LYMPHOBLASTIC LEUKEMIA

This is another lymphoblastic disease with putative viral etiology. The question of whether acute lymphoblastic leukemia is clonal or the result of cell recruitment has been debated for many years. Thus far, G-6-PD studies in acute leukemia patients have not been reported, but information relevant to this question is found in studies of the fate of marrow engrafted into leukemia recipients. In 2 patients given supralethal whole-body irradiation before marrow engraftment from histocompatibility-matched (HL-A and MLC), normal, opposite-sex sibs, cytogenetic studies showed that acute lymphoblastic leukemia recurred in donor cells.[44,45] Possible mechanisms underlying these recurrences in donor cells have been discussed,[44,45] but perhaps the most likely is that hitherto normal donor cells were recruited to form the recurrent leukemia by activation of a leukemogenic virus in donor cells or by transfer of such an agent from host to donor cells. Irradiation has been shown to activate leukemogenic virus in rodents[46] and possibly a similar activation occurred in the irradiated patients treated with marrow grafts. Fortunately, since the initial observations in these 2 patients, no further cases of leukemia relapse in donor cells have been reported.

SUMMARY

Genetic marker systems have been employed to investigate the origin and development of many human tumors. The type of information already gained with such systems includes the probable single cell origin of chronic myelocytic leukemia in a marrow stem cell. The G-6-PD system has also confirmed the hypothesis that at least some hereditary and viral tumors have multiple cell origin. However, Burkitt lymphoma, the malignancy in man for which there is a great amount of circumstantial evidence for a viral cancer, has a clonal origin. Of particular interest is the demonstration that early relapses after remissions of Burkitt lymphoma represent reemergence of the original malignant cell lines, whereas some late recurrences may be the result of newly induced malignant clones. Similarly, some recurrences of acute lymphoblastic leukemia in patients treated with marrow transplantation may be new occurrences of disease. These observations have important implications for the etiology and pathogenesis of Burkitt lymphoma and acute lymphoblastic leukemia.

REFERENCES

1. Mårtensson, L.: On a "key point of modern biochemical genetics." Lancet 1: 946, 1963.
2. Linder, D. and Gartler, S. M.: Glucose-6-phosphate dehydrogenase mosaicism: Utilization as a cell marker in the study of leiomyomas. Science 150:67, 1965.

3. Fialkow, P. J.: The origin and development of human tumors studied with cell markers. N. Engl. J. Med. 291:26, 1974.

4. Fialkow, P. J.: Use of genetic markers to study cellular origin and development of tumors in human females. Adv. Cancer Res. 15:191, 1972.

5. Rowley, J. D.: A new consistent chromosomal abnormality in chronic myelogenous leukaemia identified by quinacrine fluorescence and Giemsa staining. Nature 243:290, 1973.

6. Cannellos, G. P. and Whang-Peng, J.: Philadelphia-chromosome-positive preleukaemic state. Lancet 2:1227, 1972.

7. Fialkow, P. J., Gartler, S. M. and Yoshida, A.: Clonal origin of chronic myelocytic leukemia in man. Proc. Natl. Acad. Sci. USA 58:1468, 1967.

8. Barr , R. D. and Fialkow, P. J.: Clonal origin of chronic myelocytic leukemia. N. Engl. J. Med. 289:307, 1973.

9. Fialkow, P. J. and Jacobson, R.: Unpublished.

10. Fialkow, P. J.: Primordial cell popl size and lineage relationships of five human cell types. Ann. Hum. Genet. 37:39, 1973.

11. Fialkow, P. J., Lisker, R., Detter, J. et al: 6-Phosphogluconate dehydrogenase: Hemizygous manifestation in a patient with leukemia. Science 163:194, 1969.

12. Fialkow, P. J., Lisker, R., Giblett, E. R. et al: Genetic markers in chronic myelocytic leukaemia: Evidence opposing autosomal inactivation and favouring 6-PGD-Rh linkage. Ann. Hum. Genet. 35:321, 1972.

13. Fitzgerald, P. H., Pickering, A. F. and Eiby, J. R.: Clonal origin of the Philadelphia chromosome and chronic myeloid leukaemia: Evidence from a sex chromosome mosaic. Br. J. Haemat. 21:473, 1971.

14. Gahrton, G., Lindsten, J. and Zech, L.: Clonal origin of the Philadelphia chromosome from either the paternal or the maternal chromosome number 22. Blood 43:837, 1974.

15. Hayata, I., Kakati, S. and Sandberg, A. A.: On the monoclonal origin of chronic myelocytic leukemia. Proc. Jap. Acad. 50:381, 1974.

16. Moore, M. A. S., Ekert, H., Fitzgerald, M. G. and Carmichael, A.: Evidence for the clonal origin of chronic myeloid leukemia from a sex chromosome mosaic: Clinical, cytogenetic, and marrow culture studies. Blood 43:15, 1974.

17. Hossfeld, D. K.: Additional chromosomal indication for the unicellular origin of chronic myelocytic leukemia. Z. Krebsforsch. (In press.)

18. Clein, G. P. and Flemans, R. J.: Involvement of the erythroid series in blastic crisis of chronic myeloid leukaemia: Further evidence for the presence of Philadelphia chromosome in erythroblasts. Br. J. Haemat. 12:754, 1966.

19. Rastrick, J. M., Fitzgerald, P. H. and Gunz, F. W.: Direct evidence for presence of Ph[1] chromosome in erythroid cells. Br. Med. J. 1:96, 1968.

20. Chervenick, P. A., Ellis, L. D., Pan, S. F. and Lawson, A. L.: Human leukemic cells: In vitro growth of colonies containing the Philadelphia (Ph[1]) chromosome. Science 174:1134, 1971.

21. Finney, R., McDonald, G. A., Baikie, A. G. and Douglas, A. S.: Chronic granulocytic leukemia with Ph[1] negative cells in bone marrow and a ten year remission after Busulphan hypoplasia. Br. J. Haemat. 23:283, 1972.

22. Berger, R.: Chromsomes et leucémies humaines, la notion d'evolution clonale. Ann. Genet. 8:70, 1965.

23. de Grouchy, J., de Nava, C., Cantu, J. M. et al: Models for clonal evolution: A study of chronic myelogenous leukemia. Am. J. Hum. Genet. 18:485, 1966.

24. Motomura, S., Ogi, K. and Horie, M.: Monoclonal origin of acute transformation of chronic myelogenous leukemia. Acta Haematol. 49:300, 1973.

25. Fialkow, P. J., Sagebiel, R. W., Gartler, S. M. and Rimoin, D. L.: Mutliple cell origin of hereditary neurofibromas. N. Engl. J. Med. 284:298, 1971.

26. Schenkein, I., Bueker, E. D., Helson, L. et al: Increased nerve-growth-stimulating activity in disseminated neurofibromatosis. N. Engl. J. Med. 290:613, 1974.

27. Gartler, S. M., Ziprkowski, L., Krakowski, A. et al: Glucose-6-phosphate dehydrogenase mosaicism as a tracer in the study of hereditary multiple trichoepithelioma. Am. J. Hum. Genet. 18:282, 1966.

28. Friedman, J. and Fialkow, P. J.: Submitted for publication.

29. Murrary, R. F., Hobbs, J. and Payne, B.: Possible clonal origin of common warts (verruca vulgaris). Nature 232:51, 1971.

30. Old, L. J., Boyse, E. A., Oettgen, H. E. et al: Precipitating antibody in human serum to an antigen present in cultured Burkitt's lymphoma cells. Proc. Natl. Acad. Sci. USA 56:1699, 1966.

31. de Schryver, A., Friberg, A., Klein, G. et al: Epstein-Barr virus-associated antibody patterns in carcinoma of the postnasal space. Clin. Exp. Immunol 5:443, 1969.

32. Henle, W., Henle, G., Ho, H. C., et al: Antibodies to Esptein-Barr virus in naso-pharyngeal carcinoma, other head and neck neoplasms, and control groups. J. Natl. Cancer Inst. 44:225, 1970.

33. zur Hausen, H., Schultz-Holthausen, H., Klein, G. et al: EBV DNA in biopsies of Burkitt tumors and anaplastic carcinomas of the nasopharynx. Nature 228:1056, 1970.

34. Reedman, B. M., Klein, G., Pope, J. H. et al: Epstein-Barr virus-associated complement fixing and nuclear antigens in Burkitt's lymphoma biopsies. Int. J. Cancer 13:755, 1974.

35. Pagano, J. S., Huang, C. H. and Levine, P.: Absence of Epstein-Barr viral DNA in American Burkitt's lymphoma. N. Engl. J. Med. 289:1395, 1973.

36. Nonoyama, M., Kawai, Y., Huang, C. H. et al: Epstein-Barr virus DNA in Hodgkin's disease, American Burkitt's lymphoma, and other human tumors. Cancer Res. 34: 1228, 1974.

37. Fialkow, P. J., Klein, G., Gartler, S. M. and Clifford, P.: Clonal origin for individual Burkitt tumours. Lancet 1:384, 1970.

38. Fialkow, P. J., Klein, E., Klein, G. et al: Immunoglobulin and G-6-PD as markers of cellular origin in Burkitt lymphoma. J. Exp. Med. 138:89, 1973.

39. Fialkow, P. J., Klein, G. and Singh, S.: Unpublished observations.

40. Manolov, G. and Manolova, Y.: Marker band in one chromosome 14 from Burkitt lymphomas. Nature 237:33, 1972.

41. Clifford, P., Singh, S., Stjernswärd, J. and Klein, G.: Long-term survival of patients with Burkitt's lymphoma: An assessment of treatment and other factors which may relate to survival. Cancer Res. 27:2578, 1967.

42. Ziegler, J. L., Bluming, A. Z., Fass, L. and Morrow, R. H., Jr.: Relapse patterns in Burkitt's lymphoma. Cancer Res. 32:1267, 1972.

43. Fialkow, P. J., Klein, G. and Clifford, P.: Second malignant clone underlying a Burkitt-tumour exacerbation. Lancet 2:629, 1972.

44. Fialkow, P. J., Thomas, E. D., Bryant, J. I. and Neiman, P. E.: Leukemic transformation of engrafted human marrow cells in vivo. Lancet 1:251, 1971.

45. Thomas, E. D., Bryant, J. I., Buckner, C. D. et al: Leukaemic transformation of engrafted human marrow cells in vivo. Lancet 1:1310, 1972.

46. Kaplan, H. S.: On the natural history of the murine leukemias: Presidential address. Cancer Res. 27:1325, 1967.

Malignant Disease in Heterozygous Carriers

Michael Swift, MD

Although the frequent occurrence of skin malignancies in patients with xeroderma pigmentosum was known for many years,[1] the unusually high incidence of cancer and leukemia in other autosomal recessive syndromes was not noted until the late 1950s and 1960s (Table 1).[2-6] Along with the reports of malignant neoplasms in affected homozygous patients, there were occasional reports of malignant neoplasms occurring in young relatives who did not have the same recessive syndrome.[2,3] If they carried the gene for the syndrome, the close relatives with a malignancy had to be heterozygous. Our interest in measuring the predisposition to malignant neoplasms that might be associated with heterozygosity for a gene for one of these autosomal recessive syndromes was stimulated by estimates of heterozygote frequencies, which suggested that carriers of these genes might represent a substantial proportion of cancer patients in the general population (Table 2).

Homozygous individuals with the syndrome called Fanconi anemia (FA) are usually easily recognized by multiple diverse malformations, growth retardation, and the development of pancytopenia during childhood, adolescence, or early adult life.[7] The finding of café-au-lait spots or other abnormal skin pigmentation is frequently helpful on clinical examination, and the diagnosis of FA may be confirmed by the presence of frequent chromosome breaks and rearrangements in the lymphocyte or fibroblast cultures derived from these patients.[7]

We chose to study the extended family of each homozygous proband, since it was obvious that the available sample of obligatory heterozygotes, the parents of the patients, would be inadequate to demonstrate even a substantial increase in risk of malignancy for FA heterozygotes. Each blood relative of a patient with an autosomal recessive syndrome has, based on his relationship to the proband, a specific prior probability of being heterozygous for the gene for that syndrome

Birth Defects: Original Article Series, Volume XII, Number 1, pages 133–144
© 1976 The National Foundation

TABLE 1. Types of Malignant Neoplasms Observed in Patients with Autosomal Recessive Syndromes

Fanconi anemia	Ataxia-telangiectasia	Xeroderma pigmentosum
Acute leukemia	Acute lymphatic leukemia	Skin basal and squamous
Squamous cell carcinoma	Lymphoma	cell carcinoma
of esophagus	Dysgerminoma	Malignant melanoma
Carcinoma of skin of	Gastric carcinoma	Ocular malignancies
the anus	Glioma	Acute lymphatic leukemia
Hepatoma	Medulloblastoma	Sarcoma of testis
	Chronic lymphocytic leukemia	Carcinoma of tongue
Werner syndrome	**Bloom syndrome**	**Chediak-Higashi syndrome**
Sarcomas	Acute myeloid leukemia	Lymphoma-like phase
Meningioma	Carcinoma of tongue	Hodgkin disease
Hepatoma		
Breast carcinoma		
Thyroid carcinoma		
Acute myelogenous		
leukemia		

TABLE 2. Estimates of the Heterozygote Frequency for the Autosomal Recessive Syndromes Associated with Cancer and Leukemia

Syndromes	Approximate Incidence	Estimated Heterozygote Frequency*
Ataxia-telangiectasia	1/40,000	.01
Bloom syndrome	In Ashkenazi Jews	.005 (?)
Chediak-Higashi syndrome	?	?
Fanconi anemia	1/360,000	.003
Werner syndrome	$1-22/10^6$	.002–.09
Xeroderma pigmentosum	$1-4/10^6$	.002–.004

*Estimates of the frequency of homozygous individuals are taken from published reports[1,4,5,8,10] or from unpublished observations made in the course of our clinical studies. The frequency of heterozygotes is estimated in each case by the Hardy-Weinberg principle: if q is the frequency of the rare allele causing the syndrome and p is the frequency of the normal allele at the same locus, then $p + q = 1$ and $p^2 + 2pq + q^2 = 1$. The heterozygote frequency, $2pq$, is approximately twice q, since p is almost one, and q is estimated simply by taking the square root of the observed incidence of homozygotes, which is q^2 in the above formulation.

(Fig. 1). A significant increase in deaths from malignant neoplasms (25 observed, 15.6 expected; $p < .05$) was found in 8 families of patients with FA.[8]

We applied similar principles of data collection and analysis in our next study in which we analyzed the incidence of malignant neoplasms in the families of 27

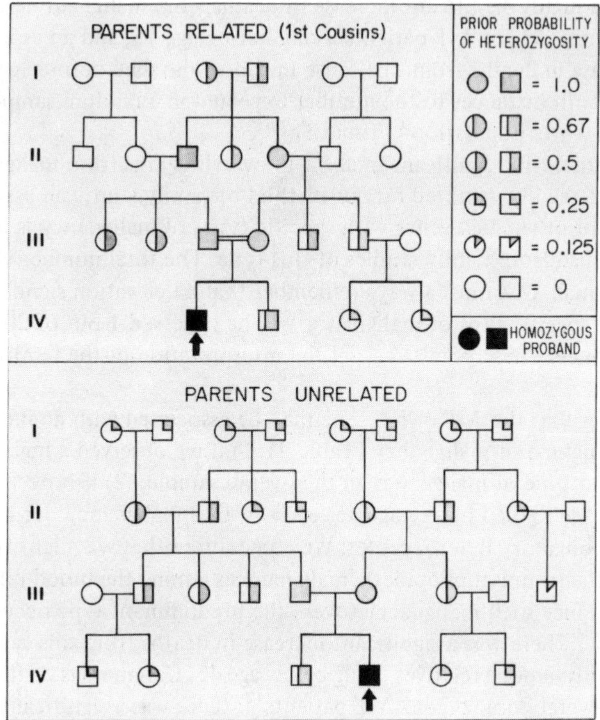

Fig. 1. The prior probability that a relative of a proband with a rare autosomal recessive syndrome will be heterozygous for the gene is proportional to the grey-shaded portion of each circle or square. These probabilities of heterozygosity are based solely on the relationship to the homozygous proband and disregard the small probability of carrying the gene as a random member of the general population. (From Swift, M., Cohen, J. and Pinkham, R.: A maximum likelihood method for the disease predisposition of heterozygotes. Am. J. Hum. Genet. 26:304, 1974, with permission of the publisher, The University of Chicago Press.)

patients with ataxia-telangiectasia (A-T).[9] This is the commonest autosomal recessive syndrome for which an association with malignancy has been recognized. Homozygous patients with this condition occur about once in every 40,000 births.[10] The clinical signs of cerebellar dysfunction and of increased susceptibility to bacterial infections when present, usually appear before the characteristic telangiectasia which may be seen on the conjunctiva, the face or ears, and in the antecubital fossa. In our experience, an increase in the serum alpha-fetoprotein[11] is a much more consistent laboratory abnormality than the decrease in the immunoglobulins which was described early in association with A-T.[12]

We found a highly significant increase in deaths from malignant neoplasms among blood relatives of A-T patients dying before age 75, and an especially striking increase in deaths from this cause in those who died before age 45, when compared in both instances to the number expected in a random sample of the United States white population[9] (Table 3).

While a statistically significant increase in overall deaths from malignant neoplasms may be readily detected by our method of family study, an association of the FA, A-T, or other such genes with specific types of malignancy is more difficult to establish from family studies of this type. The total number of observed neoplasms is small. One must always remember that an elevation significant at the 5% level for a specific type of malignancy will be observed 1 out of 20 times simply by chance. These points restrict the interpretation of the family data we have gathered.

We consider that the A-T or FA gene may be associated with an increased risk for a particular type of malignancy (Table 4) 1) if we observed a highly significant increase in that type of malignancy in the overall sample; 2) if it occurred in blood relatives who died before age 45; or 3) if that malignancy occurred in one or more of the obligatory heterozygotes. We conjectured that we might find an increase in deaths from lymphopoietic malignancies among the blood relatives of A-T patients, since such malignancies were the predominant type occurring in homozygotes.[3] There was a significant increase in deaths from this type of malignancy only among relatives dying below age 45. Carcinomas of the ovary have occurred in several homozygous A-T patients[12]; there was a significant increase in this tumor type among younger female A-T blood relatives. It was totally

TABLE 3. Deaths from Malignant Neoplasms in 27 Families of A-T Patients

	Observed*	Expected*
	From all causes	
	329	330.3
	From malignant neoplasms	
Dying ≤ 45 years	15	5.2 (p < .001)
Dying ≤ 75 years	59	42.6 (p < .02)
All ages	67	52.6
.25 probability of heterozygosity	39	37.0
.5 probability of heterozygosity	25	14.5
1.0 probability of heterozygosity	3	1.2
0.0 (spouse controls)	11	20.5

*The observed numbers of deaths from malignant neoplasm are based on the underlying cause of death recorded on death certificates, while the expected numbers for each category were obtained by applying age-race-sex-calendar-specific mortality rates to the population over the period January 1, 1903–December 31, 1974.

TABLE 4. Specific Malignancies Which May be Associated With the
A-T Gene in Heterozygotes

Type of Malignancy	In Statistical Excess	In Obligatory Heterozygotes	In Persons Dying ≤ 45 Years
Stomach	?	X	X
Large intestine		X	X
Biliary system	X		X
Basal cell		X	
Breast		X	X
Cervix		X	X
Ovary	X		X
Lymphopoietic	X	X	X

unexpected that among the 329 deaths of blood relatives 5 were due to primary carcinomas of the biliary system, a rare site of malignancy. Gastric carcinomas have occurred in homozygous A-T patients.[13] The fact, that the increase in deaths among A-T blood relatives from this cancer was not statistically significant, may be explained by the several instances in which persons who had documented carcinoma of the stomach were certified as dying from other causes.

While the data for the FA families are much more limited, it is interesting to compare the types of malignancies which were observed in the FA and A-T studies. Lymphopoietic malignancies were observed to be increased in both studies, and there was a general increase in gastrointestinal malignancies in the FA families. We thought it remarkable that 3 carcinomas of the base of the tongue were observed in the 102 deaths of the FA study (including one in an obligatory heterozygote), and that a small number of bladder carcinomas were reported in that study, while none were observed in the much larger A-T family study.

A principal criticism of our work is that an overall increase in deaths from malignant neoplasms or from specific neoplasms may not be due to an effect of the A-T or FA gene but to the selection of families from a population group or stratum with a generally increased predisposition to malignancy or to specific types of malignancies. For example, we cannot include in our study sample families disorganized by social or emotional stress. It might be true that, while the families we studied came from all social classes except the very lowest, they had received superior medical care, and that a malignant neoplasm was diagnosed as the cause of death more frequently than expected in a random sample of the general population.

To test this alternative hypothesis, we collected information about the illnesses and causes of death for nonblood relatives in the A-T families, the spouses of blood relatives in the study. In general, these spouse controls came from the same ethnic and social strata as blood relatives and were subject, for the most of their adult lives, to the same environmental influences as the blood relatives. Among the spouse controls there were significantly fewer deaths from cancer and leukemia than would be expected in the random sample of the general population (Table 3). These data provide no support for the hypothesis that our families came from a population stratum predisposed to deaths from malignancy (from factors apart from the A-T gene) and, indeed, suggest the opposite.

The data in Table 3 provide additional support for the hypothesis that the observed increase in deaths from malignant neoplasms in the A-T families was associated with the A-T gene and did not result from other familial or environmental factors. The ratio of observed to expected deaths from cancer and leukemia is greater for the blood relatives whose probability of having the A-T gene is higher (0.5 or 1.0) than for those of lower (0.25) probability of heterozygosity.

The concept of relative risk best summarizes these observations of an increased number of deaths from malignant neoplasms in the families of patients with a particular autosomal recessive syndrome. Since the study sample contains relatives whose probability of being heterozygous for the A-T or FA gene is less than one, it is not possible to estimate the relative risk for an A-T or FA heterozygote directly from the observed/expected ratio for the entire sample or for any substantial subset. We used a maximum likelihood method[14] which weights the data according to the prior probability of heterozygosity (Fig. 1) to estimate for FA or A-T heterozygotes the relative risk of dying from a malignant neoplasm.

The estimates of relative risk for the A-T or FA heterozygote of dying from a malignant neoplasm are given in Table 5. These risk estimates were used in counseling the families at the completion of our study. Such counseling can be of practical value, since many of the malignancies in the A-T or FA families are amenable

TABLE 5. Estimates of the Relative Risk of Dying From a Malignant Neoplasm for FA and A-T Heterozygotes*

	Male	Female
FA		
(all ages)	3.3	2.7
A-T		
(dying before age 45)	5.6	5.7
(dying between ages		
45 and 75)	1.8	2.2

*Relative risk estimates obtained by a maximum likelihood method[14] comparing the observed death rates from malignant neoplasm to 1950 age-race-sex-specific rates for the United States population.

to medical or surgical cure if detected and treated early enough. It is important in conveying this risk of information to the families of homozygous patients to strike a middle ground between excessive alarm and cancerphobia on the one hand and insufficient alertness on the other. Because of the parents' concern for their affected child or children and the physical and emotional costs of the child's genetic illness, it is entirely possible that a parent will ignore clear early signs of a malignancy and tragically delay seeking medical attention until there is no hope of definitive treatment. We have observed such an instance.

The product of the relative risk and the heterozygote frequency for a particular gene provides an estimate of the proportion of malignancies in the general population that may be associated with that gene (Table 6). While there are a number of inferential steps underlying such estimates, the available data suggest that over 5% of all persons dying from any malignancy before age 45 may carry the gene for A-T. Thus, each gene for an autosomal recessive syndrome which is

TABLE 6. Estimates of Relative Risk and of the Proportion of FA or A-T Heterozygotes Among All Persons Dying from Cancer or Leukemia*

Type of Malignancy	Estimate of Relative Risk	Estimated Proportion of FA or A-T Heterozygotes Among All Persons With That Malignancy
	Fanconi anemia (estimated heterozygote frequency .0033)	
All	3	.01
Acute leukemia	12	.04
	Ataxia-telangiectasia (estimated heterozygote frequency .01)	
All	2	.02
All (≤ 45 years)	5.5	.055
Ovarian (≤ 55 years)	10	.1
Lymphopoietic (≤ 45 years)	7	.07
Gastric (≤ 75 years)	8	.08
Biliary system	6	.06
Other autosomal recessive syndromes associated with malignancy		?

*The heterozygote frequency was estimated from the observed homozygote frequency according to the Hardy-Weinberg principle (see Table 2). The product of the estimated relative risk for a particular neoplasm gives an estimate of the proportion of carriers of a specific gene among all persons dying from that neoplasm.

neoplasia-predisposing in heterozygotes can be seen to be associated with a small but important fraction of all genetic predisposition to malignancy. The FA gene, for example, is presently estimated to be present in 1% of all persons dying from a malignancy.[14] The proportion of genetic predisposition to cancer, lymphoma, and leukemia which may be studied through autosomal recessive syndromes is a function of the number of such syndromes associated with malignancy, and the heterozygote frequency and relative risk of malignancy for each of the genes for these syndromes.

There are other advantages to analyzing genetic predisposition to malignancy through the study of autosomal recessive syndromes. The association of a specific gene with particular types of malignancies may be most easily detected through studying the families of homozygous patients. As Table 6 shows, for individual sites or types of malignancy the proportion of persons with a particular gene (in this case, the A-T gene) may be substantial. While this observation needs further confirmation, the association of a particular gene with a specific malignancy may be important in understanding the sequence of events leading to that malignancy. For example, carcinomas of the base of the tongue are strikingly increased in FA families, and biliary system and ovarian tumors among the relatives of A-T patients. The cellular action of an oncogenic virus or carcinogenic compound, suspected of causing one of these neoplasms, might be demonstrable only if cells carrying the FA or A-T gene were used in the relevant laboratory investigations.

The metabolic action of neoplasia-predisposing genes identified through autosomal recessive syndromes may be studied in cells derived from the homozygous individuals. Although it may be difficult to completely analyze the metabolic defect associated with A-T or FA it is still many times easier to analyze a metabolic variant in homozygotes than in heterozygotes. One useful consequence of metabolic studies of the autosomal recessive syndromes associated with malignancy would be the development of a definitive test for the heterozygote for each gene. Such a test would be useful for directly measuring the risk of cancer or leukemia in heterozygotes using established methods for measuring such risk and, eventually, in screening populations seeking those at risk for particular malignancies.

Although the study of autosomal recessive syndromes associated with cancer and leukemia offers exciting possibilities for understanding a proportion of human genetic predisposition to malignancy, it is important to understand the limitations of the family studies that have been described and of this overall approach to the genetics of neoplasia. The family studies are retrospective and inferences about the action of the gene in heterozygous carriers are indirect. We are restricted to population incidence rates and information about the nonblood relatives for control data, since there is no appropriate set of control families to be studied with the same methods. Each study requires about 5 person-years of effort with constant attention to family and interpersonal dynamics and to the completeness of the information compiled.

The gene for each autosomal recessive syndrome associated with malignancy may account for only 1 or 2% of all deaths from cancer or leukemia. However, it might be possible to identify a substantial proportion of neoplasia-predisposing genes through autosomal recessive syndromes, if only there were enough syndromes with an increased incidence of malignancy in the homozygote. While the list of rare autosomal dominant syndromes associated with malignant neoplasms is long and is being constantly enlarged, there have been almost no new associations of autosomal recessive syndromes with malignancy over the past 10 years.

Certain recessive syndromes known to be in this category may be difficult to study. The Werner syndrome seems to be exceptionally rare[4] and the criteria for diagnosis cannot be rigidly specified. Bloom syndrome is confined almost entirely to Ashkenazi Jews.[5] It may be an important neoplasia-predisposing gene in this ethnic group and should be studied for this reason.

We are presently studying about 30 families of patients with xeroderma pigmentosum. The interpretation of our data will be made more difficult by the clinical heterogeneity within the syndrome and by the fact that xeroderma patients fall into 5 complementation groups when the ability of their cells to repair UV irradiation is analyzed after cell hybridization.[1]

Other recognized syndromes may be helpful in understanding genetic predisposition to malignancy. Patients with the Chediak-Higashi syndrome often develop a terminal "lymphoma-like" phase.[6] One Chediak-Higashi patient was reported to have typical Hodgkin disease.[15] It is unclear whether Chediak-Higashi homozygotes are predisposed to malignancy in the same general way as FA, A-T, or Werner syndrome patients are. The incidence of the Chediak-Higashi syndrome and its ethnic distribution are unknown. The autosomal recessive syndromes, hemochromatosis and albinism, are thought to predispose to malignancy. It is well established that patients with the very rare syndrome, dyskeratosis congenita, are predisposed to squamous cell carcinoma and there are reports of acute lymphatic leukemia in young relatives.[16] While this syndrome seems to be exceptionally rare, only a few instances of parental consanguinity have been reported. Almost all reported cases have occurred in males and there are no examples of parent-child transmission. The mode of inheritance of this condition is uncertain, but the condition is probably X-linked recessive in most families.

Thus, while autosomal recessive syndromes may serve to designate some of the important neoplasia-predisposing genes in man, the list of such syndromes associated with malignancy is presently quite small. Perhaps some of the genes which could be identified through recessive syndromes are missed because the homozygotes do not live long enough for a malignancy to develop. For these genes, it might be possible to suspect an association of the gene with malignancy if there were an unusually high incidence of malignancies in the parents of the affected children. Clinical observations of this type should be followed by systematic family studies to determine more accurately whether the gene does predispose to cancer and leukemia.

For other syndromes, clinicians observing a single instance of malignancy occurring in a patient homozygous for a recessive condition may not think the case worth reporting; however, even single cases of malignant disease in patients with a recessive syndrome may be important, if the association of malignancy in general or of that specific malignancy with the syndrome is not well established. Alternatively, such cases should be called to the attention of investigators active in this field. We would be happy to receive such reports and to compile them for general use.

One important point to remember is using autosomal recessive syndromes to identify genes, which are relatively common and neoplasia-predisposing, is that most of the documented familial associations of malignancies are site-specific. Families of breast cancer patients show an increased incidence of this tumor type but not of malignancies generally.[17] The same is true for colonic and gastric carcinomas,[18] and for malignancies of other organs or systems. The autosomal recessive syndromes studied to date do not identify predisposition to a specific malignancy, although the FA and A-T genes are associated with an increased risk for a limited number of types of tumors.

There are theoretic and practical considerations which may be helpful in analyzing site-specific predisposition to cancer through autosomal recessive syndromes. For a gene which predisposes in the heterozygous state to a malignancy or group of malignancies, there are logically only 3 possibilites for the homozygote: 1) lethal in utero; 2) clinically normal, perhaps with a greatly increased predisposition to that malignancy or set of malignancies; or 3) clinically distinctive, ie expressed as an autosomal recessive syndrome.

For breast cancer, for example, the latter 2 possibilities could be approached in several ways. If the gene for a particular autosomal recessive syndrome predisposed the heterozygote to breast cancer, this association might be recognized by noting the appearance of an usually high incidence of this malignancy in the mothers, normal sibs, or other close maternal and paternal blood relatives of the proband. The probands themselves might not survive to the age of risk for breast cancer. A gene which predisposed to breast cancer but produces no recognizable abnormalities in homozygotes might be identified through studying the families of women whose breast carcinomas appeared at a relatively young age. If these women were predisposed to the unfortunate early onset of this tumor by a double dose of a gene which produced a smaller but measurable effect in heterozygotes, the incidence of breast cancer should be elevated among maternal and paternal blood relatives. Unless there were parental consanguinity, it would be impossible to know through family studies of this type whether the genes predisposing to breast cancer on the maternal and paternal sides were identical, at the same locus but dissimilar, or at different loci.

Autosomal recessive syndromes can be used to identify other disease-predisposing genes which are numerically important in the general population. It has already been pointed out that this approach could be used to identify genes which predispose to diabetes mellitus.[19] Moreover, the detection of genes which protect against the development of malignant disease might, in principle, be based on family studies of autosomal recessive syndromes. While the identification of genes associated with a decreased risk of malignancy would be of great importance in understanding metabolic defenses against oncogenesis, methods for selecting particular syndromes to investigate for this characteristic are not obvious at this time.

Based on the studies already completed, we recommend the following:
1) Try to identify additional autosomal recessive syndromes associated with neoplastic disease by reporting or collecting
   a) single instances in homozygotes;
   b) occurrences of malignancy in young parents of homozygotes.
2) Compile accurate information about the incidence, ethnic distribution, and parental consanguinity rate for each of the autosomal recessive syndromes which predispose to malignancy.
3) Continue family studies of autosomal recessive syndromes associated with malignant neoplasms in the homozygote.
4) Intensify metabolic studies (in homozygous cell cultures) of those genes which clinically have been shown to predispose the heterozygote to malignant disease.

The proportion of genetic predisposition to cancer and leukemia which can be analyzed through autosomal recessive syndromes depends on the number of syndromes for which the association between the syndrome and malignant disease can be established. Progress in this area depends on clarifying the genetics and epidemiology of recessive syndromes associated with malignancy and on establishing new associations through the constant alertness of clinicians and geneticists.

REFERENCES

1. Robbins, J. H., Kraemer, K. H., Lutzner, M. A. et al: Xeroderma pigmentosum: An inherited disease with sun sensitivity, multiple cutaneous neoplasms, and abnormal DNA repair. Ann. Intern. Med. 80:221, 1974.
2. Garriga, S. and Crosby, W. H.: The incidence of leukemia in families of patients with hypoplasia of the marrow. Blood 14:1008, 1959.

3. Reed, W. B., Epstein, W. L., Boder, E. and Sedgwick, R.: Cutaneous manifestations of ataxia-telangiectasia. JAMA 195:746, 1966.

4. Epstein, C. J., Martin, G. M., Schultz, A. L. and Motulsky, A. G.: Werner's syndrome: A review of its symptomatology, natural history, pathologic features, genetics and relationship to the natural aging process. Medicine 45:177, 1966.

5. German, J.: Bloom's syndrome: I. Genetical and clinical observations in the first twenty-seven patients. Am. J. Hum. Genet. 21:196, 1969.

6. Blume, R. S. and Wolff, S. M.: The Chediak-Higashi syndrome: Studies in four patients and a review of the literature. Medicine 51:247, 1972.

7. Swift, M. R. and Hirschhorn, K.: Fanconi's anemia: Inherited susceptibility to chromosome breakage in various tissues. Ann. Intern. Med. 65:247, 1972.

8. Swift, M.: Fanconi's anemia in the genetics of neoplasia. Nature 230:370, 1971.

9. Swift, M., Sholman, L., Perry, M. and Chase, C.: Malignant neoplasms in the families of patients with ataxia-telangiectasia. Cancer Res. (In press.)

10. Sedgwick, R. P. and Boder, E.: Ataxia-telangiectasia: In Vinken, P. J. and Bruyn, G. W. (eds.): "Handbook of Clinical Neurology: The Phakomatoses." New York: American Elsevier Publishing Co., Inc., 1973, vol. 14, p. 267.

11. Waldmann, T. A. and McIntire, K. R.: Serum-alpha-fetoprotein levels in patients with ataxia-telangiectasia. Lancet 2:1112, 1972.

12. Dunn, H. G., Meuwissen, H., Livingstone, C. S. and Pump, K. K.: Ataxia-telangiectasia. Can. Med. Assoc. J. 91:1106, 1964.

13. Haerer, A. F., Jackson, J. F. and Evers, C. G.: Ataxia-telangiectasia with gastric adenocarcinoma. JAMA 210:1884, 1969.

14. Swift, M., Cohen, J. and Pinkham, R.: A maximum likelihood method for the disease predisposition of heterozygotes. Am. J. Hum. Genet. 26:304, 1974.

15. Tan, C., Etcubanas, E., Lieberman, P. et al: Chediak-Higashi syndrome in a child with Hodgkin's disease. Am. J. Dis. Child. 121:135, 1971.

16. Addison, M. and Rice, M. S.: The association of dyskeratosis congenita and Fanconi's syndrome. Med. J. Aust. 1:797, 1965.

17. Macklin, M. T.: Comparison of the number of breast-cancer deaths observed in relatives of breast-cancer patients, and the number expected on the basis of mortality rates. J. Natl. Cancer Inst. 22:927, 1959.

18. Macklin, M. T.: Inheritance of cancer of the stomach and large intestine in man. J. Natl. Cancer Inst. 24:551, 1960.

19. Swift, M., Sholman, L. and Gilmour, D.: Diabetes mellitus and the gene for Fanconi's anemia. Science 178:308, 1972.

Carcinoma of the Pancreas in Four Brothers *

Jan M. Friedman, MD † and Philip J. Fialkow, MD

Although carcinoma of the pancreas is the fourth leading cause of death from cancer in the United States,[1] familial occurrence of this malignancy is rare. This report of pancreatic carcinoma in 4 brothers suggests that hereditary factors may sometimes be important in the pathogenesis of this disease.

CASE REPORTS

The proband sought genetic counseling in 1970 because his father and 2 paternal uncles had died of carcinoma of the pancreas (Fig. 1). At age 66, the proband's father, *III-6*, presented with a 2-year history of abdominal discomfort and with left infraumbilical tenderness. On laparotomy, a carcinoma of the pancreas with diffuse metastasis to the liver was found and confirmed histologically on liver biopsy material. The patient died 2 months later.

III-5, an uncle of the proband, at age 67 developed epigastric pain and anorexia. He was found to be markedly emaciated and to have a fixed right upper quadrant abdominal mass. Surgical exploration revealed carcinoma of the body of the pancreas with extensive metastasis to the liver and pelvis. Histologic examination of a liver biopsy specimen confirmed this diagnosis. The patient died a few weeks later.

A second uncle, *III-4*, presented at age 66 with acute pain and marked tenderness in the right upper quadrant of his abdomen. At surgery, there was a 600–700 ml hemoperitoneum and a large tumor in the head and body of the pancreas. The liver contained many metastatic nodules, one of which was biopsied to confirm the diagnosis. The patient expired in 4 weeks.

*This work was aided by USPHS grant GM 15253.

†Awarded Public Health Service fellowship F22-CA03128

Birth Defects: Original Article Series, Volume XII, Number 1, pages 145–150

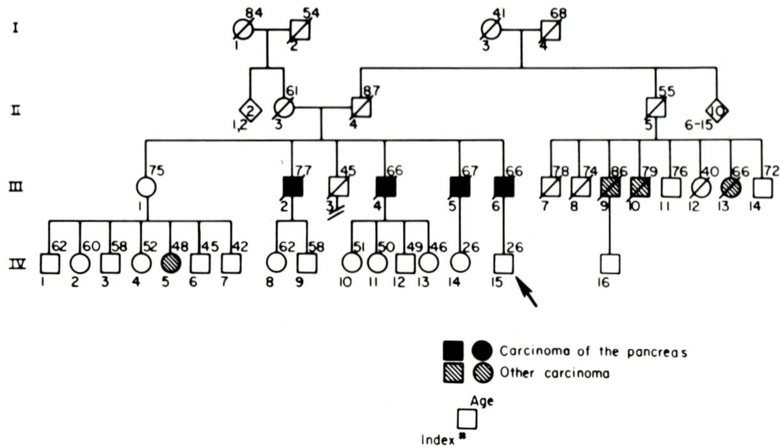

Fig. 1. Family pedigree, including 4 brothers with pancreatic carcinoma.

In 1975, 4½ years after the proband's first Genetics Clinic visit, carcinoma of the pancreas was diagnosed in a third uncle, *III-2*. This 77-year-old man had chronic obstructive lung disease, chronic peptic ulcer disease, and a 3-year history of mild diabetes mellitus. His present illness consisted of 6 weeks of jaundice, weakness, and anorexia. On physical examination, he appeared cachectic and deeply icteric. A large, cystic mass was palpated in the right upper quadrant of his abdomen. On exploratory laparotomy, the gall bladder was found to be greatly distended. A 5—6 cm firm, multilobulated mass was present in the head of the pancreas. No evidence of metastasis was seen, but the tumor was felt to be unresectable and was not biopsied. The patient died 6 weeks later.

In none of the 4 affected brothers was an autopsy performed. In the 3 in whom biopsies were obtained, the histologic character of the tumor varied from completely undifferentiated carcinoma to mucinous adenocarcinoma (Figs. 2—4).

The only living member of the sibship is a sister, *III-1*, who is now in her 70s (Fig. 1). Her daughter, *IV-5*, had a cervical carcinoma resected at 35 years of age. The other male in the affected sibship, *III-3*, died at age 45 of pneumonia. Their mother, the proband's grandmother, *II-3*, died at age 61 during gall bladder surgery. No further information concerning her illness is available. The proband's grandfather, *II-4*, died of a myocardial infarction at age 87. One of his brothers had 3 children who developed cancer: a son, *III-9*, who died with adenocarcinoma of the prostate at 86 years of age, a daughter, *III-13*, who died at age 66 of adenocarcinoma of the ascending colon, and another son, *III-10*, who had a papillary adenocarcinoma of the rectum resected at age 64 and an adenocarcinoma of the prostate removed at 78 years of age. Both tumors were histologically proven. No other family member is known to have had a malignancy and none has a history suggestive of pancreatitis. The family is of Western European descent and denies consanguinity.

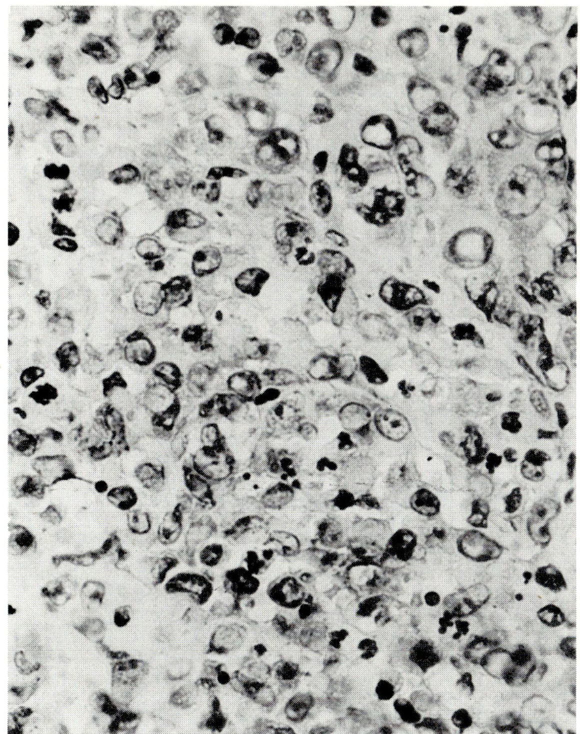

Fig. 2. Liver biopsy specimen from *III-4* showing very anaplastic carcinoma (× 360).

DISCUSSION

Although the pancreas is a relatively frequent site of involvement in patients who die of cancer in this country,[2] the probability that 4 sibs developed this malignancy by chance alone is extremely remote — about 1 in 10^9. Furthermore, since pancreatic carcinoma was diagnosed in the fourth brother after the family had been identified, ascertainment bias is unlikely.

Hereditary pancreatitis is known to predispose to carcinoma of the pancreas.[3-5] In such families, this malignancy is occasionally seen even in persons without clinical pancreatitis.[4] No member of our family had symptoms or surgical findings suggestive of pancreatitis. Furthermore, pancreatic calcification, a common sign in hereditary pancreatitis, was not noted in any of these patients with pancreatic carcinoma on abdominal radiologic examination.

Cancer of the pancreas has also been reported in association with "Cancer Families."[6,7] Patients with this syndrome, as in others with a simple inherited predispostion to tumors, are characterized by unusually early onset of malignancy

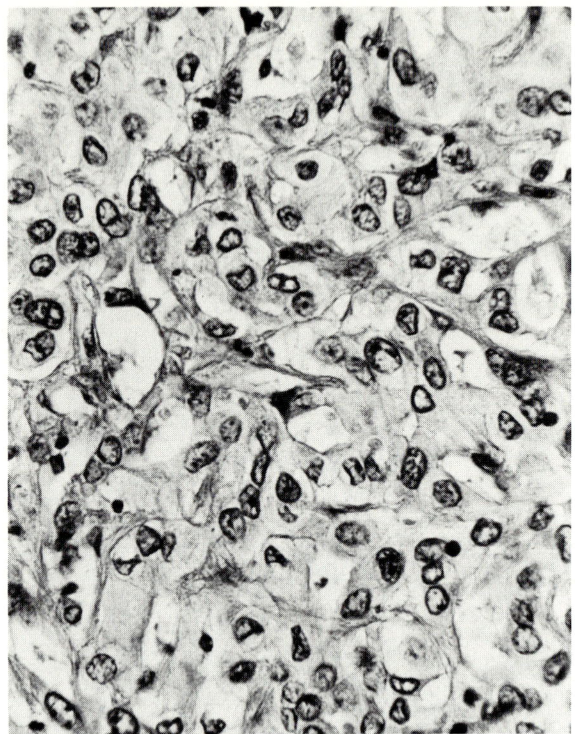

Fig. 3. Liver biopsy specimen from *III-5* showing mucinous adenocarcinoma (× 360).

and by multiple primary neoplasms.[8] In our family, carcinomas did not occur at an early age, and only one elderly gentleman had 2 tumors, both of very frequently involved sites (rectum and prostate).

Common exposure to a strong carcinogen specific for the pancreas could account for the occurrence of pancreatic cancer in these 4 brothers, all of whom worked in the logging industry. Although an association between carcinoma of the pancreas and certain occupations has been suggested,[9] no association between logging and this malignancy was found in a recent study of the causes of death of lumbermen.[10]

MacDermott and Kramer described a similar family in which 3 brothers and a sister developed carcinoma of the pancreas between the ages of 69 and 72.[11] The data from these 2 families suggest that an hereditary predisposition to pancreatic cancer late in life can occur. It is unclear whether this predisposition is transmitted in a monogenic or polygenic fashion. Moreover, it is uncertain what effect, if any, environmental factors may have played in the development of these cancers.

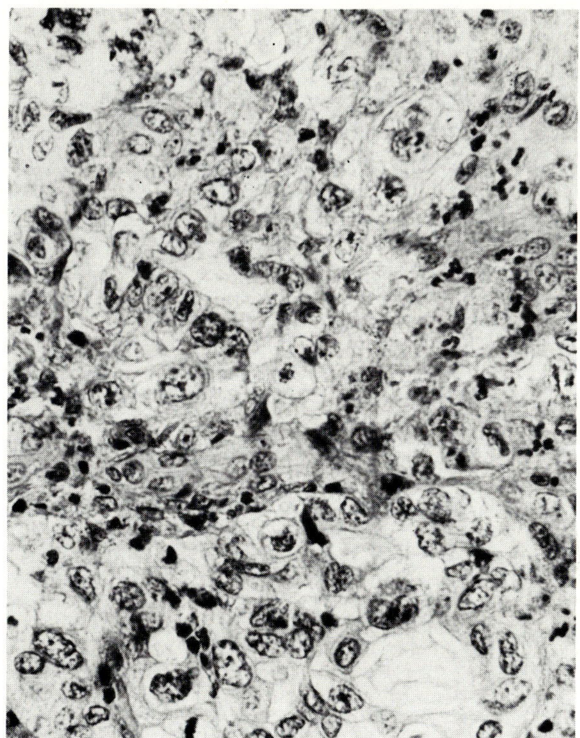

Fig. 4. Liver biopsy specimen from *III-6* showing poorly differentiated adenocarcinoma (× 360).

ACKNOWLEDGMENTS

The authors are grateful to Ms. Roberta Power for her assistance with this investigation, to Dr. Fred Smith for allowing us to study his patient, and to Dr. George Martin for reviewing the histopathology.

REFERENCES

1. Cancer statistics, 1975. CA 25:8–21, 1975.
2. Levin, D.L. and Connelly, R.R.: Cancer of the pancreas: Available epidemiologic information and its implications. Cancer 31:1231–1236, 1973.
3. Gross, J.B., Ulrich, J. A. and Maher, F. T.: Further observations on the hereditary form of pancreatitis. In deReuck, A.V.S. and Cameron, M.P. (eds.): "Ciba Foundation Symposium on the Exocrine Pancreas, Normal and Abnormal Functions," Boston: Little Brown, 1962, pp. 278–309.
4. Case records of the Massachusetts General Hospital: Case 25–1972. N. Engl. J. Med. 286:1353–1359, 1972.

5. Kattwinkel, J., Lapey, A., diSant'Angese, P. A. and Edwards, W. A.: Hereditary pancreatitis: Three new kindreds and a critical review of the literature. Pediatrics 51:55–69, 1973.

6. Lynch, H.T.: "Cancer families": Adenocarcinomas (endometrial and colon carcinoma) and multiple primary malignant neoplasms. Recent Results Cancer. Res. 12:125–142, 1967.

7. Li, F.P. and Fraumeni, J.F.: Soft-tissue sarcomas, breast cancer, and other neoplasms – a family syndrome? Ann. Intern. Med. 71:747–752, 1969.

8. Knudson, A.G., Strong, L. C. and Anderson, D. E.: Heredity and cancer in man. Prog. Med. Genet. 9:113–158, 1973.

9. Wynder, E.L., Mabuchi, K., Maruchi, N. and Fortner, J. G.: Epidemiology of cancer of the pancreas. J. Natl. Cancer Inst. 50:645–667, 1973.

10. Milham, S.: Personal communication.

11. MacDermott, R.P. and Kramer, P.: Adenocarcinoma of the pancreas in four siblings. Gastroenterology 65:137–139, 1973.

Familial Reticulum Cell Sarcoma*

Victor Escobar, DDS and David Bixler, PhD, DDS

INTRODUCTION

With the notable exception of monogenic syndromes involving cancerous and precancerous disorders,[1] it is evident from the literature that there are certain families which are unusually prone to the development of malignancy.[1-11] Furthermore, there appear to be reported familial cases of lymphoma in which the authors have emphasized the hereditary aspects in tumor production,[7,8,12-14] while others have emphasized the role of environment as a causative agent.[3,4,15,16] Lynch has suggested that for certain cancers we might be dealing with 2 kinds of families: 1) Anatomic site-specific or tumor-specific families, and 2) Non-anatomic site-specific families.[17] This classification of families has resulted in the delineation of the cancer family syndrome.[1,18] Pedigrees of families with this syndrome clearly show that the incidence of cancer is increased remarkably among family members, and there is an apparent dominant transmission pattern to the syndrome. In addition, there is a significantly increased incidence of multiple primary malignancies in the affected individuals.[9,10,19] It is obvious then, that multiple anatomic-site families fit this syndrome very well, whereas the anatomic site-specific or single type tumor families[5,6] do not fit the definition completely. On these grounds, one may assume that different genotypes are responsible for the phenotypes in both types of families, eg genetic heterogeneity exists for this trait.

Genetic heterogeneity is a concept which supports the idea that the lymphomas constitute distinct clinical entities and this has been proposed for familial primary upper small intestinal lymphoma.[2] However, evidence is accumulating

*This is publication number 75–15 from the Medical Genetics Department and was supported in part by the Indiana University Human Genetics Center PHS P 01 GM 21054 and by a LASPAU Fellowship.

Birth Defects: Original Article Series, Volume XII, Number 1, pages 151–158

that environmental factors also play a significant role in the production of that entity, especially in view of the geographic distribution of the disease.[20-23]

Previous reports of familial occurrences of lymphomas are summarized in Table 1. These lymphomas usually occurred in site-specific families and followed dominant[14] or recessive[15,24,25] patterns of inheritance. Indirect proof that genetic factors are involved in the production of familial lymphoma is found in the familial association of disorders of the immune system and lymphomas.[4,26] Further support is presented by Fuller,[27] who observed that patients suffering lymphomas had dermatoglyphic patterns differing signficantly from those in control groups.

In postulating a familial predisposition to lymphoma one must take into account that this is a heterogeneous disease category and the fact that several members of a family have suffered from this disease may be coincidence. Furthermore, it is important to recall the recent discovery of a human tumor virus which was isolated from patients with leukemia.[28]

The purpose of this report is to describe a "cancer family" in which all affected individuals had the occurrence of reticulum cell sarcoma (RCS) in common. To our knowledge this is the first reported family in which RCS has occurred in direct lineage and in which RCS appeared in 6 successive generations.

TABLE 1. Summary of Previous Reports of Familial Lymphoma

| Author | Proband | | | Relationship | Lesion | Inheritance |
	Sex	Age	Lesion			
Banihashemi[2]	F	22	Leukemia	Brother (28y)	RCS	AR?
	M	6½	RCS	Brother (18y)	RCS	AR?
Hambleton[7]	M	4½	Lympho-sarcoma	Brother (3½y)	Lympho-sarcoma	AR?
Johnson[8]	M		Leukemia	3 Sibs	Leukemia Sarcoma	AR?
Miller[25]	M	1 mo	RCS	4 Sibs (ly)	RCS	AR
Potolsky[15]	M	67	Lympho-sarcoma	4 Sibs	Leukemia	
				1 Sib	RCS	AR?
				1 Sib	Carcinoma	
Rigby[14]	M	63	Multiple myeloma	Sister (68y)	RCS	AD?
				Niece (38y)	Leukemia	
				Grandson (4y)	Leukemia	
Takats[16]	F	68	Leukemia	Husband (73y)	RCS	
	F	74	Leukemia	Husband (77y)	RCS	

AR = Autosomal Recessive
AD = Autosomal Dominant
RCS = Reticulum Cell Sarcoma
Y = Age in years

CASE HISTORY AND RESULTS

The proband (*III-10*) was a 74-year-old, caucasian, diabetic female admitted
to Indiana University Hospital with a 6-month history of pain in the epigastric
region, which started while eating and lasted 1½–2 hours. Vomiting occurred
usually after meals. No hematemesis or melena were present. X-ray GI series
showed a filling defect on the greater curvature which, after abdominal exploration and subtotal gastrectomy (80%), proved histopathologically to be
RCS. Sixty days after surgery the patient developed increasing anorexia,
nausea, bloody vomiting and loss of weight; Hodgkin disease was diagnosed.
The patient died on her 4th day of hospitalization with a progressive lymphocyte pulmonary infiltration.

Her medical history revealed that 8 years previously (age 66), she had undergone a hysterectomy for carcinoma of the cervix.

Family history revealed multiple occurrences of cancer in the proband's
sibship as well as in other near relatives. The family pedigree is shown in Figure 1 and the pertinent family history is summarized in Table 2.

The total number of family members we have been able to trace is 116, of
which 13 have had multiple occurrences and recurrences of adenocarcinoma,
carcinoma and RCS. The organs involved are from multiple systems and include
larynx, lung, stomach, breast, cervix, skin, and face.

In *Generation III* of this family all 5 female sibs suffered the disease, including

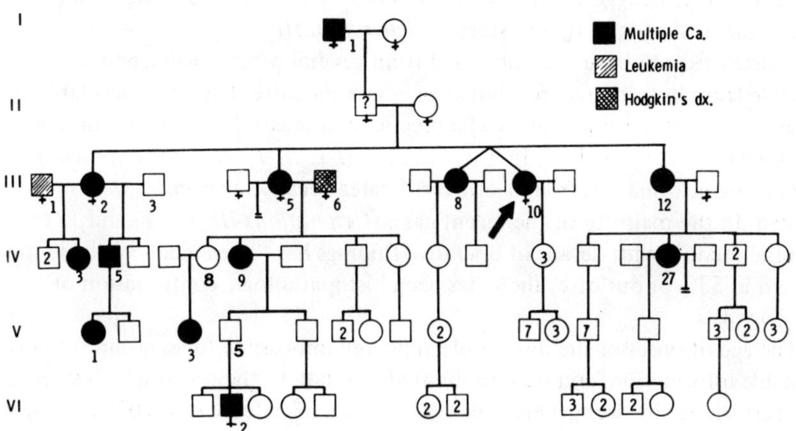

Fig. 1.

TABLE 2.

Pedigree index no.	Sex	Carcinoma	Adenocarcinoma	RCS	Age
I-1	M	?	?	?	d 51
III-1	M			Leukemia, by history	d 46
III-2	F	Larynx (67)	Breast (64)	Stomach (69)	d 70
III-5	F		Breast (71)	Liver (74)	d 74
III-6	M			Hodgkin, by history	d 71
III-8	F	Colon (46)	Endometrium (68)		75
III-10	F	Cervix (66)		Hodgkin (74) Stomach (74)	d 74
III-12	F	Fundus (58)	Pancreas (60)	Esophagus*	78
IV-3	F	Larynx (55)	Lung (59)	Lung (60)	61
IV-5	M	Basal Cell (48)		Stomach (55)*	55
IV-9	F	Breast (45)	Uterus (50)		61
IV-27	F	Squamous cell, cervix (32)		Colon (42)	55
V-1	F			Lung*	32
V-3	F	Breast (34)			41
VI-2	M			Maxillar (3)	d 3

*Patients actually in treatment.

Number in ( ) = age at diagnosis.

a pair of dizygotic twins (Table 2). Three of these females have passed the condition on to their children, grandchildren and even great-grandchildren. Also interesting and highly suggestive is the occurrence of leukemia and Hodgkin disease in 2 of the husbands of these sisters of *Generation III*.

Causes of death have been obtained from general practitioners, and where possible from hospital records, but even where the latter have been available it has not always been possible to be precise with regard to the anatomic site and type of cancer involved. In 3 of the cases (*I-1, III-1, III-6*) we have had to rely on the information from death certificates because necropsies were not performed. In the majority of the recent cases (*Generations III, IV, V, and VI*) hospital records with details of operative findings have been made available to us, and in 53% of our cases there has been histopathologic confirmation of the diagnosis.

The age of onset of the disease often proved impossible to ascertain from available information, and we have limited our data to the age at which surgery was performed. In later generations the mean age of affecteds has been younger than in earlier generations. In *Generation III*, there were 5 affected females with average age of onset of 61.6 years. In *Generation IV*, there were 4 affecteds with average age of onset of 45 years. In *Generation V*, there were 2 affected females whose average age of onset was 33 years, while in *Generation VI* there has been only a single affected (*VI-2*), a male who died at the age of 3.

Of all deaths to date in this family, 16 have been documented, of which 7 have been due to RCS, 3 to pyloric stenosis, 1 to alcoholism and 3 to heart conditions. Two more deaths have occurred, one due to Hodgkin disease and the other to leukemia. These last 2 persons were husbands of patients of *Generation III* and consequently not blood relatives.

There are 2 exceptions to regular transmission of RCS, (*IV-8* and *V-5*), indicating that reduced penetrance is present. However, it may be that these individuals, as well as other members of the family who are at risk, have not yet attained the age of onset.

A remarkably high incidence of tuberculosis has been noted both in patients with malignancies and in their families.[18, 29] *Patient V-1* suffered TB at the age of 18 and subsequently developed a malignancy of the lung at age 32.

DISCUSSION

The etiology of malignancies of the reticuloendothelial system has received a great deal of attention. This is probably due to the quest for a viral etiology to malignancies of this tissue.[28, 30] Genetic studies have received less attention, and consequently, few examples of familial lymphomas exist in the literature (Table 1). These few reports have emphasized a probable hereditary basis for malignancy of this type. If these genetic bases really exist, a strong suggestion for genetic predisposition to cancer arises. Proof for this genetic predisposition must await studies of family members who have been environmentally separated.

The rarity of lymphomas, even among members of families with affected individuals suggests a genetic predisposition, which if present does not correspond to a simple mode of inheritance. However, considering our present understanding of cancer etiology, we should not reject the genetic hypothesis, even when aspects of familial lymphoma may well be representations of environmental factors as suggested in previous reports.[20–23] If the hypothesis of environmental factors is to hold true, the individuals must be in the proper environment at a susceptible time. Studies from France and Israel[8] suggest that this susceptible time may be infancy and the environmental factors may be repeated viral infections and possible altered immune mechanisms. However, even when these studies are postulating an environmental agent as the main cause of the disease, they still refer to a genetic mechanism (immune system deficiencies) as responsible in large part for the production of the disease.

We are fortunate to have available to us a large kindred in whom pathologic verification of tumors has been obtained, but of unusual interest is the increased occurrence of RCS in this kindred. The occurrence of reticuloendothelial neoplasms is in sharp distinction to neoplasms observed in the cancer family syndrome[1] in which there has been an excess of adenocarcinoma and carcinoma. The dominant inheritance pattern also differentiates this family from other reports of familial lymphoma in which the transmission of the disease apparently has been recessive.[8, 14, 20]

Because of the rarity of familial RCS the following explanation is considered for its occurrence: A genetic predisposition to cancer that appears to have a simple mode of inheritance is present in this family. This has been reported for other types of tumors[2, 5, 6] but never for RCS.

If this hypothesis is true, what we might be observing in this kindred is the genetic segregation of a gene defect in the process of information transfer.[31] This information transfer allows for alterations among genes required for normal differentiation.[32] Disruption of this mechanism might result in the production of cancer without the presence of an oncogenic virus.

A second alternative to consider in this family is the transmission of a viral genome mimicking genetic transmission. Genetic studies in mice[33] show that this is not an untenable hypothesis. Investigators working with malignant human cells have frequently observed virus-like particles in those cells.[28] They also have observed extensive homologies between DNA tumor viruses, as well as antigens similar to those present in animal viruses.[30] This evidence has convinced many that viruses are involved in human cancer, but identification of the viruses themselves has remained elusive. Several publications have attempted to relate breast cancer and B-RNA tumor viruses, a type that in animals has been associated exclusively with mammary tumors.[34] Leukemia has also been associated with viruses. However the leukemia virus is a type of C-RNA tumor virus, which is the most common class of animal tumor viruses. Type C-RNA tumor viruses have also been implicated in the production of lymphomas and sarcomas. As in leukemia, human breast cancer has been consistently demonstrated to show familial aggregation,[35] but epidemiologic evidence provides no support for a viral etiology. In the same way, there is no epidemiologic evidence in support of a viral etiology for human lymphomas, although some familial aggregation may occur.[8, 12, 14, 17] Furthermore, neither of the known human viruses has been proven to be a causative agent in human tumors.

Perhaps a viral genome has been integrated into one of the chromosomes of the host, thereby explaining the transmission of susceptibility from one generation to the next. Onset of cancer in a member of this family may be related to conversion of the virus from the temperate to the lysogenic stage.

In summary, it is impossible to choose between the etiologic hypotheses. We are examining biopsy and surgical tissue by EM studies in the hope of identifying a viral genome, and thereby provide concrete evidence in favor of a viral etiology.

REFERENCES

1. Lynch, H. and Krush, A. J.: Differential diagnosis of the cancer family syndrome. Surg. Gynecol. Obstet. 136:221–224, 1973.
2. Banihashemi, A., Najr, K., Heydayattee, H. and Mortazave, E.: Familial lymphoma including a report of a familial primary upper small intestinal lymphoma. Blut 26: 363–368, 1973.
3. Bracha, R. and Many, A.: Primary intestinal lymphoma: Clinical manifestations and possible effect of environmental factors. Recent Results Cancer Res. 39:193–199, 1972.
4. Creagan, E. T. and Fraumeni, J. F.: Familial gastric cancer and immunological abnormalities. Cancer 32:1325–1331, 1973.
5. Dunstone, G. H. and Knaggs, T. W.: Familial cancer of the colon and rectum. J. Med. Genet. 9:451–454, 1972.
6. Epstein, L., Bixler, D. and Bennett, J.: An incident of familial cancer. Cancer 25: 889–891, 1970.
7. Hambleton, G. and Gotton, D. G.: Familial lymphoma. Proc. R. Soc. Med. 62:1095–1099, 1969.
8. Johnson, M. J., Peters, C. H. and Bismark, N. D.: Lymphoma in four siblings. JAMA 1: 63–167, 1957.
9. Lynch, H. and Krush, A. J.: Family "G" revisted, 1895–1970. Cancer 27:1505–1511, 1971.
10. Lynch, H., Krush, A. J. and Guirgis, H.: Genetic factors in families with combined gastrointestinal and breast cancer. Am. J. Gastroenterol. 59:31–40, 1973.
11. Lynch, H., Krush, A. J., Harlan, W. and Sharp, E. A.: Association of soft tissue sarcoma, leukemia and brain tumors in families affected with breast cancer. Am. Surg. 39:199–206, 1973.
12. Borden, E. C.: Viruses and breast cancer. Implications of mouse and human studies. Johns Hopkins Med. J. 134:66–76, 1964.
13. Rigby, P. G., Papenfuss, H. L. and Lennon, H. M.: Familial lymphoma. J. Lancet 86:379–384, 1966.
14. Rigby, P. G., Prat, P., Roseula, J. R. and Lemon, H.: Genetic relationships in familial leukemia and lymphoma. Arch. Intern. Med. 121:67–69, 1967.
15. Potolsky, A. I., Hrath, C. W., Buckley, C. E. and Rowlands, D. J.: Lymphoreticular malignancies and immunologic abnormalities in a sibship. Am. J. Med. 50:42–48, 1971.
16. Takats, L. J. and Csapo, Z.: Malignant lymphomas occurring in marital partners. Case reports on two couples. Br. J. Cancer 22:173–175, 1968.
17. Lynch, H., Krush, A. J. and Larsen, A. L.: Hereditary and endometrial carcinoma. South. Med. J. 60:231–235, 1967.
18. Lynch, H., Shaw, M. W., Magnuson, C. et al: Hereditary factors in cancer: Study of two large midwestern kindreds. Arch. Intern. Med. 117:206–212, 1966.
19. Lynch, H.: Hereditary factors in carcinoma. Recent Results Cancer Res. 12:125–142, 1967.
20. Dutz, W., Asvadi, S. and Hohout, E.: Intestinal lymphoma and spine. Gut 12:804, 1971.
21. Eidelman, S., Parkins, R. and Rubin, C.: Abdominal lymphosarcoma presenting as malabsorption. Medicine (Baltimore) 45:111–116, 1966.

22. Gleinsenger, M. H., Ahmy, T. P. and Barr, D. P.: The sprue syndromes secondary to lymphoma of the small bowel. Am. J. Med. 15:666, 1953.
23. Ramot, B.: Malabsorption due to lymphomatous disease. Annu. Rev. Med. 22: 19–21, 1971.
24. Givler, R.: Lymphocyte leukemia with coexisting localized RCS. Cancer 21:1184– 1192, 1968.
25. Miller, D. R.: Familial reticuloendotheliosis – concurrence of disease in five siblings. Pediatrics 38:986–995, 1966.
26. Tsuji, K., Ito, M., Miyamoto, H. and Yamashita, H.: HL-A antigenic loss in a cancer patient, a case report. Gann 63:495–497, 1972.
27. Fuller, U. C.: Inherited predisposition to cancer? A dermatoglyphic study. Br. J. Cancer 28:186–189, 1973.
28. Maugh, T.: Leukemia: A second human tumor virus. Science 187:335–336, 1975.
29. Lynch, H.: History of cancer genetics in man. Recent Results Cancer Res. 12: 18–20, 1967.
30. Sherr, E. and Todaro, G.: Primate type C virus p30 antigens in cells from humans with acute leukemia. Science 187:855–856, 1975.
31. Temin, H. M.: The protovirus hypothesis: Speculation on the significance of RNA-directed DNA synthesis for normal development and for carcinogenesis. J. Natl. Cancer Inst. 46(2):3–7, 1971.
32. Allen, D. and Cole, P.: Viruses and human cancer. N. Engl. J. Med. 286:70–82, 1972.
33. Chang, S. S. and Hiderman, W. H.: Inheritance of susceptibility to polyoma virus in mice. J. Natl. Cancer Inst. 33:303–313, 1964.
34. Chopra, H. C. and Mason, M. M.: A new virus in a spontaneous mammary tumor of a rhesus monkey. Cancer Res. 30:2081–2086, 1970.
35. MacDermott, R. D. and Kramer, P.: Adenocarcinoma of the pancreas in four siblings. Gastroenterology 65:137–139, 1973.

Possible Linear Order of Genes for Endocrine Neoplasia Type 2, the P Red Cell Antigen and HL-A on Chromosome 6[*]

Charles E. Jackson, MD, P. Michael Conneally, PhD,
Glen W. Sizemore, MD, and Armen H. Tashjian, Jr., MD

Two autosomal dominantly inherited endocrine neoplasia syndromes have been delineated on the basis of clinical features.[1] The glands involved in type 1 consist of the parathyroids, pancreatic islets and the pituitary with most cases of hereditary hyperparathyroidism being a part of this syndrome.[2,3] In type 2, the parathyroid glands are involved in association with medullary carcinoma of the thyroid (MCT) and adrenal pheochromocytomas.[1] A possible variant[4,5] of type 2 occurring with similar glandular involvement in association with mucosa neuromas and/or the marfanoid habitus has been termed 2b and also termed type 3.[6]

Linkage investigations of 2 large families with MCT (*SLA* and *STA* kindreds previously reported[7]) have been combined with the screening for affected members utilizing calcium[7,8] and pentagastrin[9,10] provocative tests for calcitonin secretion. Utilizing these provocative test procedures the penetrance of the gene for MCT is thought to be quite high, probably in the teens, especially if the premalignant stage of "C cell hyperplasia" is included.[7,11] In the larger family with 25 affected members (*SLA* kindred), HL-A typing was performed on all available individuals (Fig. 1). The *STA* kindred is shown schematically in Figure 2. For the 2 families a total of 2 recombinants and 14 nonrecombinants was found in the P vs MCT linkage analysis. Mayo Clinic kindred *KOE* has been informative in the P-MCT relationship with 2 recombinants and 4 nonrecombinants in offspring of an affected female. Eleven recombinants and 15 nonrecombinants were found in the HL-A vs MCT linkage analysis (Fig. 1). Further linkage

*This study has been supported in part by USPHS grants AM 14876, AM 10206 and AM 21054.

Birth Defects: Original Article Series, Volume XII, Number 1, pages 159—164

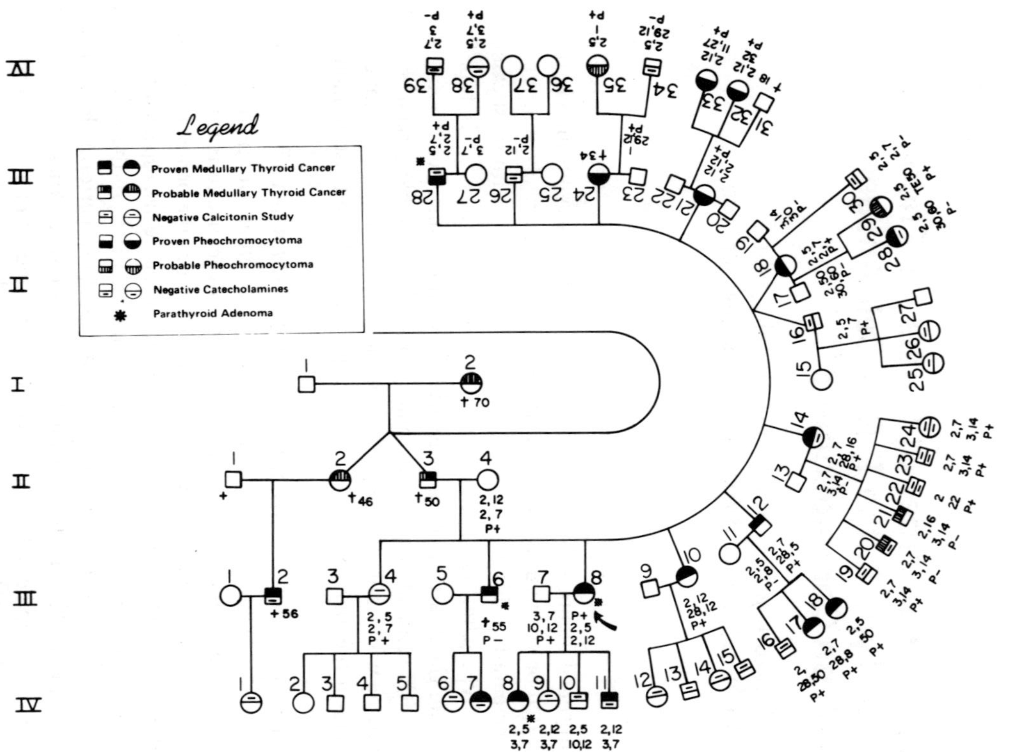

Fig. 1. *SLA* kindred modified from reference 7 to provide HL-A and P data and information on 4 additional members found to be affected. The following individuals have negative calcitonin studies but are probably too young yet for this test to be considered reliable: *IV-19, IV-24, IV-38, and IV-39.* The 2,16 haplotype in individual *III-14* is thought to be a mutation.

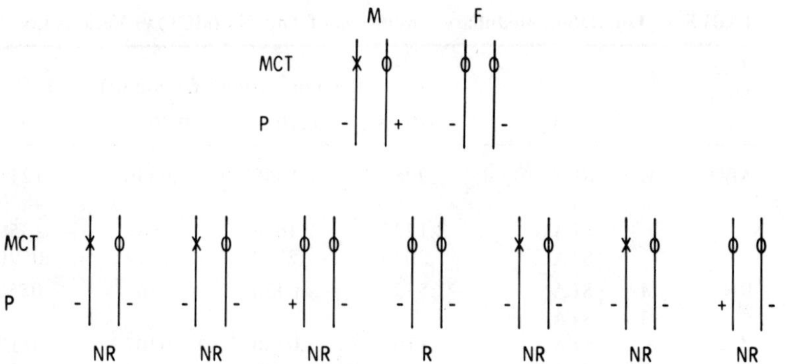

Fig. 2. *STA* kindred modified from reference 7 to illustrate schematically the theorized P red cell typing and the affected status.

analysis performed to provide lod scores for these relationships has not provided assurance of the P-MCT linkage (Table 1). The program LIPED written by Ott[12] was used to compute lod scores for males and females for each family separately. The program analyzes the family as a unit, thus obtaining maximum information on the recombination fraction in contrast to some other methods which can only analyze a sibship at a time. The program also finds inconsistencies in the family. Since the trait is extremely rare it has been assumed that no individual marrying into the family carries the trait. Close linkage with the MCT locus (Table 1) can be excluded for ABO, Rh, MNS, acid phosphatase and HL-A $(\theta < -2.0)$.

The P antigen and HL-A have been reported to be loosely linked[13] but further data suggest that this may be dubious.[14-16] The HL-A locus is thought to be located on chromosome 6.[17] If the present data suggesting that the MCT locus may be linked to the P antigen locus can be confirmed, the evidence that the MCT locus is distant to the HL-A locus would provide an estimate of the linear order on chromosome 6 of the genes for these conditions (if P should be proved to be linked even loosely to HL-A). We are pursuing linkage studies of the endocrine neoplasia syndrome with other loci such as PGM_3 reported[18] to be on chromosome 6.

Studies of families of the mucosal neuroma phenotype of the medullary thyroid carcinoma-pheochromocytoma syndrome (Mayo Clinic *THO* kindred) have been so far uninformative regarding P linkage. If the P-MCT linkage is confirmed in other studies, the finding of no close linkage of the mucosal neuroma syndrome with P would provide evidence that this syndrome is an entity separate from the usual endocrine neoplasia type 2 syndrome. Likewise, if the mucosal neuroma phenotype were found to be linked to a locus to which the usual type 2 phenotype were clearly unlinked, further evidence would be

TABLE 1. Lod Scores Medullary Carcinoma of Thyroid (MCT) vs Various Loci*

Loci MCT vs	Sex	Family	Recombination Fraction (θ)			
			0.10	0.20	0.30	0.40
ABO	M	SLA	− .9957	− .1869	.0890	.1241
	M	STA	−	−	−	−
	F	SLA	−3.1727	−1.4046	− .5581	− .1350
	F	STA	− .3079	− .2082	− .1272	− .0590
RH	M	SLA	−1.5124	− .6490	− .2461	− .0555
	M	STA	−	−	−	−
	F	SLA	.1106	.0780	.0407	.0112
	F	STA	−2.0969	−1.1938	− .6655	− .2907
MNS	M	SLA	−1.7079	− .5609	− .0863	.0697
	M	STA	−1.3980	− .7959	− .4437	− .1938
	F	SLA	− .9916	− .4432	− .1752	− .0413
	F	STA	−1.3311	− .5815	− .2272	− .0532
Kidd	M	SLA	− .1103	− .0511	− .0206	− .0054
	M	STA	− .2448	− .14461	− .0768	− .0305
	F	SLA	− .3897	− .1821	− .0776	− .0223
	F	STA	− .3717	− .1334	− .0327	− .0049
Duffy	M	SLA	− .0962	− .0692	− .0417	− .0181
	M	STA	.0211	.0146	.0089	.0040
	F	SLA	− .0649	.1630	.2104	.1508
	F	STA	.0099	.0075	.0045	.0017
P	M	SLA	− .5929	− .2788	− .1156	− .0294
	M	STA	−	−	−	−
	F	SLA	.0332	.1883	.1457	.0395
	F	STA	.5316	.5262	.3601	.1309
AcP	M	SLA	−1.1419	− .5903	− .2966	− .1143
	M	STA	−	−	−	−
	F	SLA	−3.5558	−1.7148	− .7874	− .2639
	F	STA	−1.3311	− .5815	− .2216	− .0532
ADA	M	SLA	0.0	0.0	0.0	0.0
	M	STA	−	−	−	−
	F	SLA	0.0	0.0	0.0	0.0
	F	STA	−1.5195	− .5712	− .1568	− .0083
HP	M	SLA	−0.0002	0.0001	0.0001	0.0
	M	STA	−	−	−	−
	F	SLA	− .0595	− .0325	− .0141	− .0035
	F	STA	− .0182	− .0595	.0342	.0059
HL-A	M	SLA	−3.2771	−1.5116	− .6536	− .1975
	M	STA	−	−	−	−
	F	SLA	−1.4527	− .3567	.0598	.1489
	F	STA	−	−	−	−

*Lod scores for θ linkage of medullary carcinoma of the thyroid vs various loci (LIPED program utilized at Indiana University Department of Medical Genetics[12]).

provided for the 2 conditions being separate entities. The rapid progress being made at present in gene linkage relationships will allow the delineation of more and more clinical conditions on the basis of chromosome linkage.

ACKNOWLEDGMENTS

The authors gratefully acknowledge the assistance of Dr. H. Hayashi and Ms. M. Guenther for the HL-A studies, Dr. S. Saeed for blood group studies, Ms. Joann Yott for genetic field work, Mrs. Nancy Nielsen for the red cell and serum protein polymorphism studies, and Miss Janet Tice and Miss Elizabeth Kormos for the calcitonin assays performed in Dr. Tashjian's laboratory.

REFERENCES

1. Steiner, A. L., Goodman, A. D. and Powers, S. R.: Study of a kindred with pheochromocytoma, medullary thyroid carcinoma, hyperparathyroidism and Cushing's disease: Multiple endocrine neoplasia, type 2. Medicine 47:371, 1968.
2. Jackson, C. E. and Boonstra, C. E.: The relationship of hereditary hyperparathyroidism to endocrine adenomatosis. Am. J. Med. 43:727, 1967.
3. Jackson, C. E. and Frame, B.: Relationship of hyperparathyroidism to multiple endocrine adenomatosis. In Bergsma, D. (ed.): Part X, "The Endocrine System," Birth Defects: Orig. Art. Ser., vol. VII, no. 6, Baltimore: Williams & Wilkins Co., for The National Foundation–March of Dimes, 1971, p. 66.
4. Schimke, R. N., Hartmann, W. H., Prout, T. E. and Rimoin, D. L.: Syndrome of bilateral pheochromocytoma, medullary thyroid carcinoma and multiple neuromas. N. Engl. J. Med. 279:1, 1968.
5. Gorlin, R. J., Sedano, H. O., Vickers, R. A. and Cervenka, J.: Multiple mucosal neuromas, pheochromocytoma and medullary carcinoma of the thyroid – A syndrome. Cancer 22:293, 1968.
6. Khairi, M. R. A., Dexter, R. N., Burzynski, N. J. and Johnston, C. C.: Mucosal neuroma, pheochromocytoma and medullary thyroid carcinoma: Multiple endocrine neoplasia type 3. Medicine 54:89, 1975.
7. Jackson, C. E., Tashjian, A. H., Jr. and Block, M. A.: Detection of medullary thyroid cancer by calcitonin assay in families. Ann. Intern. Med. 78:845, 1973.
8. Tashjian, A. H., Jr., Howland, B. G., Melvin, K. E. W. et al: Immunoassay of human calcitonin. Clinical measurement, relation to serum calcium and studies in patients with medullary carcinoma. N. Engl. J. Med. 283:890, 1970.
9. Hennessy, J. F., Wells, S. A., Ontjes, D. A. and Cooper, C. W.: A comparison of pentagastrin injection and calcium infusion as provocative agents for the detection of medullary carcinoma of the thyroid. J. Clin. Endocrinol. Metab. 39:487, 1974.
10. Sizemore, G. W. and Go, V. L. W.: Stimulation tests for diagnosis of medullary thyroid carcinoma. Mayo Clin. Proc. 50:53, 1975.
11. Wolfe, H. J., Melvin, K. E. W., Cervi-Skinner, S. J. et al: C-cell hyperplasia preceding medullary thyroid carcinoma. N. Engl. J. Med. 289:437, 1973.
12. Fellous, M., Billardon, C., Dausset, J. and Frezal, J.: Linkage probable entre les locus HL-A et P. C. R. Acad. Sci. (D) (Paris) 272:3356, 1971.
13. Edwards, J. H., Allen, F. H., Glenn, K. P. et al: The linkage relationships of HL-A. In "Histocompatibility Testing," Copenhagen: Munksgaard, 1972, p. 745.

14. Edwards, J. H.: Total lods for linkage analyzed by the New York Blood Center and Birmingham Computer Programs. In Bergsma, D. (ed.): "Human Gene Mapping," New Haven Conference (1973)," Birth Defects: Orig. Art. Ser., vol. X, no. 3, Miami: Symposia Specialists for The National Foundation—March of Dimes, 1974, pp. 187–189.

15. Robson, E. B.: Personal communication.

16. Borgaonkar, D. S. and Bias, W. B.: HL-A loci and chromosome 6. In "Human Gene Mapping," op. cit., pp. 67–68.

17. Lamm, L. U., Svejgaard, A. and Kissmeyer-Nielsen, F.: PGM_3: HL-A is another linkage in man. Nature (New Biol.) 231:109, 1971.

18. Ott, J.: Estimation of the recombination fraction in human pedigrees: Efficient computation of the likelihood for human linkage studies. Am. J. Hum. Genet. 26:588, 1974.

Gonadoblastoma and Dysgerminoma with Ataxia-Telangiectasia *

Marylou Buyse, MD , C. Thomas Hartman, MD and
Miriam G. Wilson, MD

Ataxia-telangiectasia (A-T), a recessively inherited syndrome affecting multiple organ systems, was described by Madame Louis-Bar[1] as a progressive cerebellar ataxia with telangiectasia of the bulbar conjunctivae and skin and frequent sinopulmonary infections. More recently, A-T has been recognized as a complex disorder with an immune deficiency, endocrinologic abnormalities and increased incidence of malignancy.[2-7] A predisposition to lymphoreticular tumors occurs in persons affected with A-T, although various other neoplasms have been reported.[8] This report describes a patient with A-T who also had a gonadoblastoma and dysgerminoma of the ovary.

CASE REPORT

A 16-year-old black female was the product of an uncomplicated term pregnancy. The birthweight was 2869 gm. She was the 7th of 12 children born to this mother. The other children in the sibship had a different father. All half-sibs were alive and well except for a younger half-sister with asthma. There was no family history of consanguinity or neurologic illness.

Early developmental stages of the proposita included the following: sitting at 7 months, independent walking at 12 months, and a vocabulary of about 10 words at 15 months. In general, speech development was slower and less distinct than that of her sibs. She was able to run and play with other children. At approximately 4 years of age she began walking on her toes and falling frequently, but she was able to attend kindergarten and first grade in a regular public school. Due to increased unsteadiness and frequent pulmonary infections, she did not attend school for the next 3 years. Following a hospitalization for pneumonia,

*This study was supported in part by USPHS grant 286 from Maternal and Child Health Services.

Birth Defects: Original Article Series, Volume XII, Number 1, pages 165—169

she was enrolled in a school for the orthopedically handicapped. By this time, she had had rubeola, mumps and varicella without sequelae. At 8 years of age, redness of the conjunctivae and jerking eye movements were noted by the parents. At 10, she was unable to walk independently but could pull up and walk holding on to furniture. An IQ score measured by a Binet test was 43. Pulmonary function was severely compromised by chronic bronchiectasis. Menarche was at age 13 with the development of normal female secondary sexual characteristics. At age 16, during a hospitalization for pneumonia, she developed nausea, vomiting and abdominal pain. She had been amenorrheic for the previous 3 months, and a weight loss of 4 kg was noted.

On *physical examination*, the proposita was a small, emaciated black female who appeared younger than her age of 16 years. Height and weight were both below the 3rd percentile for age at 127 cm and 23 kg, respectively. Her blood pressure was 100/60 mm Hg. Telangiectasia were present in the bulbar conjunctivae. A moderate degree of thoracic kyphoscoliosis was evident. Respirations were labored with rales and abdominal breathing. The fingernails were clubbed but not cyanotic. The antecubital fossae showed a coarse, desquamating, non-erythematous rash and thickened skin. A suprapubic midline mass was palpable up to the umbilicus. She had a female escutcheon, axillary hair, and mature nipple and breast development. The genitalia were normal postpubertal female. Neurologic examination revealed a slow dysarthric speech. There was a persistent bilateral left horizontal nystagmus. An intention tremor involving all limbs and truncal ataxia were present. The generalized muscular atrophy and weakness were more pronounced distally. There was no limitation of joint mobility. Deep tendon reflexes were uniformly depressed. Performance of rapid alternating movements and fine finger movement was poor. She was able to sit up from a supine position and stand from a sitting position without assistance. She could walk 10 to 15 steps with assistance.

Laboratory findings revealed that hemoglobin was 11.5 gm% and WBC was 15,300/mm^3 with an absolute lymphocyte count of 900. Plasma albumin was 3.5 gm% and globulin, 4.5 gm%. Immunoglobulins, as measured by immunodiffusion were as follows: IgG 2400 mg%, IgM 190 mg%, IgA 2 mg%, IgE 20 IU/ml. Intradermal skin tests with streptokinase-streptodornase (400 units/ml), mumps, monilia (1–10), and PPD (5 TU) were negative. Lymphocyte transformation with phytohemagglutinin was poor. A chromosome analysis from peripheral blood culture showed an apparently normal female karyotype (46,XX).

Serum human chorionic gonadotropin and alpha-fetoprotein were negative. Multiple blood glucose determinations were normal. Urine determination for ketosteroids was 2 mg/24 hrs (normal female 6–15 mg/24 hrs) and for ketogenic steroids was 5 mg/24 hrs (normal 3–15 mg/24 hrs).

An ECG was within normal limits. EEG tracing showed a mild generalized, paroxysmal irregularity. Audiologic evaluation was normal. A radiogram of the abdomen showed a large midline pelvic mass without calcification. Radiographic examination by barium enema confirmed the presence of this pelvic mass which displaced the colon. Chest, long bone and skull radiograms were normal. A bone scan showed increased uptake of radionucleotide in the right iliac wings and accumulation in the kidneys with delayed excretion. A liver scan was normal. An IVP showed bilateral hydronephrosis and hydroureter. B-scan ultrasonography suggested a 17 cm right ovarian mass.

On surgical exploration of the abdomen, a large right pelvic mass was found which contained a necrotic and hemorrhagic center. Microscopic examination of this tissue disclosed a dysgerminoma extending into the ovarian capsule and mesosalpinx (Fig. 1). Although the left ovary appeared grossly normal, biopsy from this tissue disclosed a gonadoblastoma. Both fallopian tubes were hypoplastic and the uterus was small. A bilateral salpingo-oophorectomy was performed. Six months after surgery the patient died of respiratory failure secondary to chronic bronchiectasis and pulmonary fibrosis.

Autopsy findings. Significant pathologic findings at postmortem examination were found in the respiratory, lymphatic, urogenital, endocrine and central nervous systems. Pulmonary abnormalities consisted of multiple pleural adhesions, severe bronchiectasis and several bronchiectatic cysts. The left lung weighed 200 gm, the right 250 gm. The spleen was small (70 gm) and firm, with an indistinct follicular pattern and generalized lymphoid hypoplasia with few plasma cells on microscopic examination. There were no grossly visible lymph nodes in the axilla, groin, mediastinum or retroperitoneum; however, lymph nodes detected on microscopic examination were hypoplastic. A $3 \times 2 \times 2$ cm mass occupying the position of the left ovary consisted of soft, pale homogeneous tissue without any architectural landmarks of a normal ovary. The microscopic diagnosis of this mass was dysgerminoma. There was no evidence of metastasis. The uterus was small and infantile. The adrenals were thin and atrophic with a cortical thickness of about 1 to 2 mm bilaterally. The pituitary was grossly normal and was not examined microscopically. The cerebellum showed diffuse atrophy and, on microscopic examination, degeneration of Purkinje cells and decreased cells in the granular layer, especially in the vermis. Subependymal telangiectasia

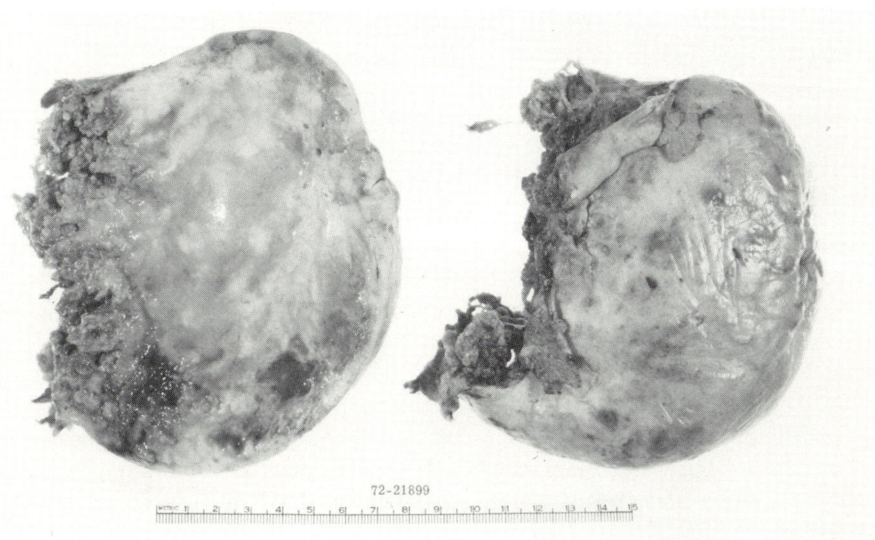

Fig. 1. Cut section, dysgerminoma.

were present in the lateral ventricles, optic chiasm and medulla. Sections of the spinal cord showed decreased numbers of anterior horn cells and slight gliosis. No definite lateral spinal column degeneration was present but pallor of myelin in the fasciculus gracilis of the cervical segments was noted. One section of low thoracic cord showed marked prominence of capillaries in both the gray matter and leptomeninges, suggesting telangiectasia.

DISCUSSION

The immunologic deficiency in A-T is frequently associated with low serum IgA, thymic hypoplasia and lymphocytopenia. The association of A-T with a defective thymus and malignancy was first described by Peterson et al[4] in 1964. The Immunodeficiency-Cancer Registry recently listed 145 persons with primary immunodeficiency disease and cancer, 52 of whom had A-T.[9] It is estimated that a person with A-T has a 10% chance of developing a malignancy.[8] Lymphoreticular tumors are most commonly found.[8,9]

Ovarian abnormalities in patients with A-T have been previously reported.[10,11] To our knowledge, the only other case of gonadal tumor with A-T was that reported by Dunn et al,[12] who described bilateral dysgerminomata in an affected child. Hypoplasia of the ovarian follicles and gonadal dysgenesis were described in conjunction with A-T.[10] It was suggested that the underlying thymic defect in this disorder may be responsible for these ovarian changes.[11] Nishizuka and Sakakura[13] were able to induce ovarian hypoplasia in female mice thymectomized on the third day of life. When thymectomy was performed later, no ovarian changes were found, and the ovarian hypoplasia could be prevented by thymic grafting. Neither control animals nor thymectomized males showed any gonadal changes. At present, the precise relationship of the thymic hypoplasia in A-T to the ovarian hypoplasia is unknown.

More information is required about the gonadal function of patients with A-T. For example, the frequency of ovarian changes in this disease is unknown since gonadal examination is not always reported. Evidently, gonadal function should be carefully evaluated in individuals with A-T since the disease may predispose to abnormal gonadal development. As evidenced by our patient, gonadal function may coexist with ovarian disease.

The association of dysgenetic gonads with germ cell tumors is well-established.[14-17] As these tumors tend to be quite small, the diagnosis of gonadoblastoma is often made only after careful microscopic examination. The malignant potential of gonadoblastoma is not established but the association of gonadoblastoma with dysgerminoma, a malignant tumor, is well-known. It has been estimated that 50% of gonadoblastomas occur with a concurrent dysgerminoma.[18] Possibly these tumors occur more frequently with A-T than now realized. The finding of both these tumors in association with A-T in the patient reported here may be yet another consequence of this extensive multisystem disorder.

REFERENCES

1. Louis-Bar, D.: Sur un syndrom progressif comprenant des télangiectasies capillaires cutanées et conjunctivales symétriques, à disposition naevoide et des troubles cérébelléux. Confin. Neurol. (Basel) 4:32, 1941.
2. Boder, E. and Sedgwick, R.P.: Ataxia-telangiectasia: A familial syndrome of progressive cerebellar ataxia, oculocutaneous telangiectasia and frequent pulmonary infection. Pediatrics 21:526, 1958.
3. Barlow, M.H., McFarlin, D.E. and Schalch, D.S.: An unusual type of diabetes mellitus with marked hyperinsulinism in patients with ataxia-telangiectasia. Clin. Res. 13:530, 1965.
4. Peterson, R.D.A., Kelly, W.D. and Good, R.A.: Ataxia-telangiectasia: Its association with a defective thymus, immunological-deficiency disease and malignancy. Lancet 1:1189, 1964.
5. Peterson, R.D.A., Cooper, M.D. and Good, R.A.: Lymphoid tissue abnormalities associated with ataxia-telangiectasia. Am. J. Med. 41:342, 1966.
6. Peterson, R.D.A. and Good, R.A.: Ataxia-telangiectasia. In Bergsma, D. (ed.): "Immunologic Deficiency Diseases in Man," Birth Defects: Orig. Art. Ser. vol. IV, no. 1. White Plains: The National Foundation-March of Dimes, 1968, p. 370.
7. Ammann, A.J., Cain, W.A., Ishizaka, K. et al: Immunoglobulin E deficiency in ataxia-telangiectasia. N. Engl. J. Med. 281:469, 1969.
8. Gatti, R.A. and Good, R.A.: Occurrence of malignancy in immunodeficiency diseases. Cancer 28:89, 1971.
9. Kersey, J.H., Spector, B.D. and Good, R.A.: Primary immunodeficiency diseases and cancer: The Immunodeficiency-Cancer Registry. Int. J. Cancer 12:333, 1973.
10. Miller, M.E. and Chatten, L.: Ovarian changes in ataxia-telangiectasia. Acta Paediat. Scand. 56:559, 1967.
11. McFarlin, D.E., Strober, W. and Waldmann, T.A.: Ataxia-telangiectasia. Medicine 51:281, 1972.
12. Dunn, H.G., Meuwissen, H., Livingston, C.S. and Pump, K.K.: Ataxia-telangiectasia. Can. Med. Assoc. J. 91:1106, 1964.
13. Nishizuka, Y. and Sakakura, T.: Thymus and reproduction: Sex-linked dysgenesis of the gonad after neonatal thymectomy in mice. Science 166:753, 1973.
14. Patel, K.K. and Prentice, R.S.A.: Gondadoblastoma, a distinctive ovarian tumor. Arch. Pathol. 94:165, 1972.
15. Talerman, A., Huyzinga, W.T. and Kuipers, T.: Dysgerminoma. Obstet. Gynecol. 41:137, 1973.
16. Schellhas, H.: Malignant potential of the dysgenetic gonad. Part I. Obstet. Gynecol. 44:298, 1974.
17. Schellhas, H.: Malignant potential of the dysgenetic gonad. Part II. Obstet. Gynecol. 44:455, 1974.
18. Scully, R.E.: Gonadoblastoma. A review of 74 cases. Cancer 25:1340, 1970.

Leukemia in a Twin with Multiple Congenital Limb Abnormalities

Juliet Hananian, MD, Kjell Koch, MD and Colin J. Condron, MD

An intriguing association exists between inherited or acquired blood disorders and skeletal limb deficiencies. The pathogenesis, however, remains unknown. A case report further illustrates this association.

A 4-year-old white female (Fig. 1) of a set of same-sex twins was born with multiple congenital anomalies consisting of right transverse hemimelia, intercalary partial radial and ulnar; bilateral paraxial fibular hemimelia of the complete longitudinal type; and bilateral ectropodia (Table 1). The remaining physical examination was normal. The first-born twin was normal. This was the 19-year-old mother's first pregnancy. Historically, she received a few antiemetic pills for vomiting early in her pregnancy.

Careful review of the mother's prenatal records revealed that she had received Provera. The birthweight of the patient was 2126 gm and the twin sister was 2466 gm. The mother's blood group is O−, both twins are O+. Complete blood group studies were obtained in another institution and the interpretation was that "the chances of their being monozygotic works out to approximately 96%."[1] Dermatoglyphic comparison for monozygosity could not be completed because of absence of the right hand in one twin. However, comparison of the left hands showed identical digital prints. A below elbow prosthesis was fitted, and when the child was 2½ years old osteotomy of the proximal right tibia was performed for progressive genu valgus deformity. Acute lymphocytic leukemia was diagnosed when the child was 2 years, 10 months old. The peripheral blood chromosome studies with and without phytohemagglutinin showed no abnormalities. Likewise, the chromosome studies of the twin sister and mother were also normal. Initially, the proband responded to antileukemia chemotherapy; however, she developed CNS leukemia and died from sepsis 3 years after the initial diagnosis of leukemia at age 6 years.

Birth Defects: Original Article Series, Volume XII, Number 1, pages 171–176

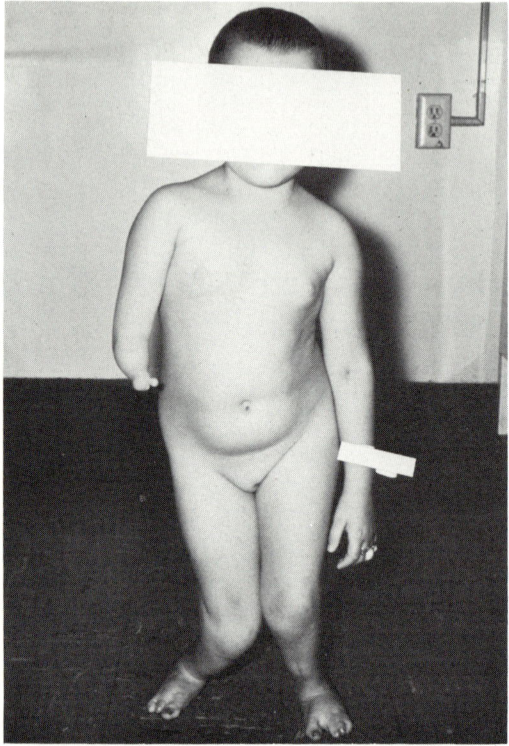

Fig. 1. The patient at age 4 years.

TABLE 1. Summary of Limb Malformations

1. Right transverse hemimelia, intercalary partial radial and ulnar
2. Bilateral paraxial fibular hemimelia complete longitudinal type
3. Bilateral hypodactyly
   Right tridactyly
   Left tetradactyly

TABLE 2. Syndromes Associated with Combined Skeletal and Blood Cell Abnormalities

1. Fanconi anemia
2. Thrombocytopenia absent radius (TAR syndrome)
3. Triphalangeal thumbs associated with hypoplastic anemia
4. Phocomelia with congenital thrombocytopenia and myeloid
   leukemoid reactions

The incidence of severe limb malformations is rare in humans, occurring approximately 1/20,000 deliveries.[2] Assuming that the incidence of acute lymphocytic leukemia in whites under 15 years of age is 4/100,000,[3] it seems unlikely that the 2 relatively rare disorders should affect the same child, particularly when the twin sister is entirely normal.

Gross malformations of limbs have been associated with maternal ingestion of thalidomide[4] and possibly haloperidol[5] in early pregnancy. Maternal diabetes and femoral aplasia or hypoplasia in the offspring have been associated on rare occasions.[6] It also occurs with some chromosome disorders and syndromes, ie Cornelia de Lange syndrome. Association of hydramnios and oligoamnios, and absence of defects of longitudinal type have been reported.[2] Recently, Janerich et al[7] in a controlled study, investigated the effects of exposure to exogenous sex steroids during pregnancy and its effects on the offspring. Their conclusion was that there is an association between exogenous sex hormones during gestation and congenital limb reduction deformities. Although this conclusion might still be debatable and controversial,[8,9] it warrants careful controlled prospective studies to further clarify the potential teratogenic effects of exogenous sex steroids. It is of interest that the mother of our patient had Provera during pregnancy, although its role in dual teratogenic and limb reduction anomalies in the patient is still unanswered.

Association of syndromes with combined skeletal defects and blood cell abnormalities are well known[10-12] (Table 2). The confirmed association is

TABLE 3. Skeletal Defects and Leukemia

Number	Skeletal Defect	Leukemia (type)	Authors
1	Marfan	AL*	Reisman[13]
1	Marfan	AL	Miller[14]
2	Osteogenesis imperfecta	ALL†	Gilchrist[15]
1	Osteogenesis imperfecta	AL	Miller[14]
1	Osteochondromatosis	AML‡	Miller[14]
1	Klippel-Feil syndrome	Congenital AML	Bernhard[16]
1	Ellis-van Creveld syndrome	Congenital AML	Miller[17]
1	Achondroplasia	ALL	Fraumeni[18]
1	Poland syndrome	ALL	Mace[19]
1	Hereditary brachydactyly	ALL	Corberland[20]
8	Fanconi anemia	AML and myelomonocytic	Dosik[21]

*AL = acute leukemia
†ALL = acute lymphocytic leukemia
‡AML = acute myelogenic leukemia

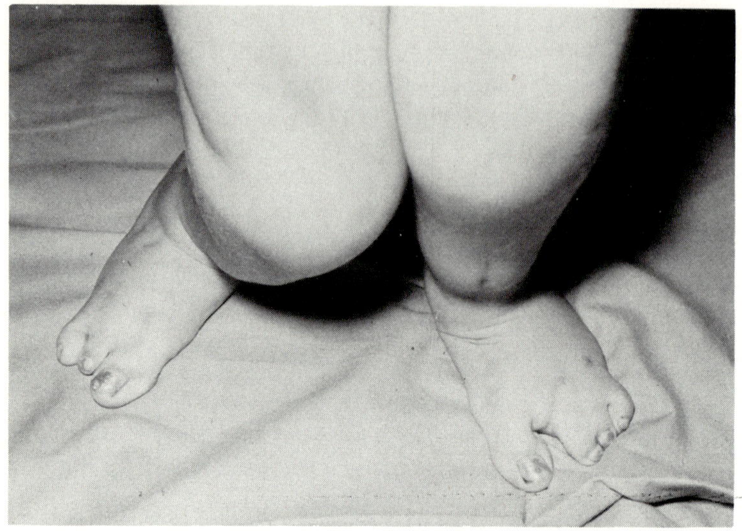

Fig. 2. Lower limbs. Flexion and valgus deformities of knees. Right tridactyly, left tetradactyly and syndactyly.

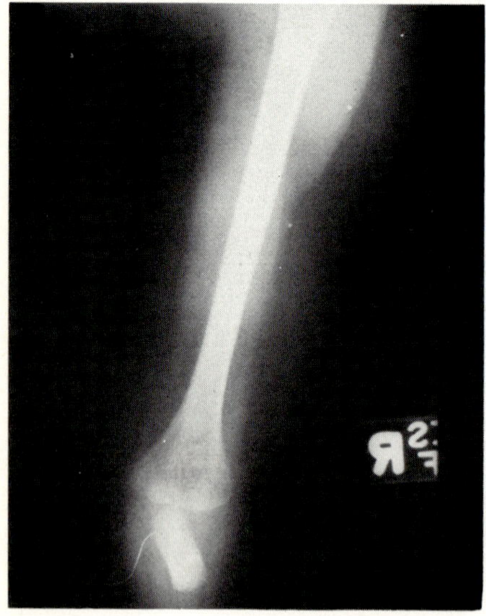

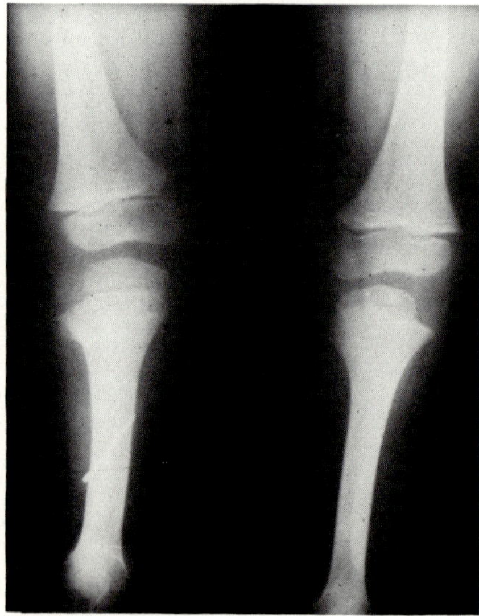

Fig. 3. X-ray picture of right upper limb. Below-elbow right transverse hemimelia.

Fig. 4. X-ray film of lower limbs. Bilateral paraxial fibular hemimelia, complete longitudinal type. Varus osteotomy right tibia.

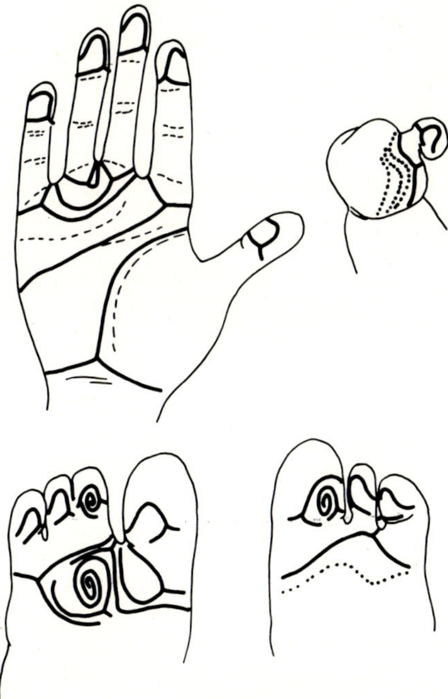

Fig. 5. Dermatoglyphics of the 6 digits showed 5 ulnar loops and one radial loop with a ridge count of 66 on the left hand. Due to a malformed right hand, the other 4 digits were missing. The *atd* angle of the left hand was 42° with the *t* triradius in a normal position. A small distal loop was present in the III interspace. The hallucal area of the right sole showed an open field with an *e* triradius, the left a large distal loop.

Fanconi anemia which is an inherited disorder, characterized by multiple congenital abnormalities, aplastic anemia, and chromosome anomalies. Patients, and possibly family members, have been noted to have an increased incidence of leukemia. A number of cases with genetically induced skeletal defects and leukemia have been reported in the literature[13–21] (Table 3).

In summary, acute lymphocytic leukemia developed in a same-sex twin who had congenital multiple limb abnormalities. Effects of maternal administration of Provera as a possible pathogenesis is unclear.

REFERENCES

1. Smith, S. M. and Penrose, L. S.: Monozygotic and dizygotic twin diagnosis. Ann. Hum. Genet. 19:273, 1955.
2. Rogala, E. J., Wynne-Davies, R., Littlejohn, A. and Gormley, J.: Congenital limb anomalies: Frequency and aetiological factors. J. Med. Genet. 11:221, 1974.
3. Young, J. L., Jr. and Miller, R. W.: Incidence of malignant tumors in U.S. children. J. Pediatr. 86:254, 1975.

4. Williams, R. T., Schumacher, H. and Smith, R. L.: The chemistry and metabolism of thalidomide. In Swingard, C. A. (ed.): "Limb Development and Deformity: Problems of Evaluation and Rehabilitation," Springfield: Charles C Thomas, 1969, chapter 5.

5. Kopelman, A. E., McCullar, F. W. and Heggeness, L.: Limb malformations following maternal use of haloperidol. JAMA 231:62, 1975.

6. Lenz, W. and Maier, W.: Congenital malformations and maternal diabetes. Lancet 2:1124, 1964.

7. Janerich, N. T., Piper, J. M. and Glebatis, D. M.: Oral contraceptives and congenital limb-reduction defects. N. Engl. J. Med. 291:697, 1974.

8. Oakley, G. P., Jr., Flynt, J. W., Jr. and Falek, A.: Hormonal pregnancy tests and congenital malformations. Lancet 2:256, 1973.

9. Clifford, R. K.: Oral contraceptives and congenital limb reduction defects. N. Engl. J. Med. 292:267, 1975.

10. Dignan, P and Mauer, A. M.: Mechanisms of myeloid leukemoid reactions associated with skeletal abnormalities. J. Pediatr. 67:939, 1965.

11. Dignan, P., Mauer, A. M. and Frantz, C.: Phocomelia with congenital hypoplastic thrombocytopenia and myeloid leukemoid reactions. J. Pediatr. 70:561, 1967.

12. Jones, B. and Thompson, H.: Triphalangeal thumbs associated with hypoplastic anemia. Pediatrics 52:609, 1973.

13. Reisman, L. E., Mitani, M. and Zuelzer, W. W.: Chromosome studies in leukemia. N. Engl. J. Med. 270:591, 1964.

14. Miller, R. W.: Childhood cancer and congenital defects: A study of U.S. death certificates during the period 1962–1966. Pediatr. Res. 3:389, 1969.

15. Gilchrist, G. S. and Shore, N. A.: Familial leukemia and osteogenesis imperfecta. J. Pediatr. 71:115, 1967.

16. Bernhard, W. G., Gore, I. and Kilby, R. A.: Congenital leukemia. Blood 6:990, 1951.

17. Miller, D. R., Newstead, G. J. and Young, L. W.: Perinatal leukemia with a possible variant of the Ellis-van Creveld syndrome. J. Pediatr. 74:300, 1969.

18. Fraumeni, J. F. and Manning, M. D.: Achondroplasia and leukemia. Br. Med. J. 3:680, 1967.

19. Mace, J. W., Kaplan, J. M., Schanberger, J. E. and Gotlin, R. W.: Poland's syndrome. Clin. Pediatr. (Phil.) 11:98, 1972.

20. Corberland, J., Rochioccioli, P., Pris, J. and Regnier, C.: Association of hereditary Type C brachydactyly and acute lymphoblastic leukemia. Ann. Pediat. 21:885, 1974.

21. Dosik, H., Hsu, L., Todaro, G. et al: Leukemia in Fanconi's anemia: Cytogenetic and tumor virus susceptibility studies. Blood 36:341, 1970.

Somatic Recombination as Possible Prelude to Malignant Transformation*

Eberhard Passarge, MD and Claus R. Bartram

Malignant transformation is heralded when a heritable somatic change leads to the development of a cell clone that differs in genetic endowment from the host.[1-4] A variety of processes have been proposed as the original event. Ohno[3] postulated the expression of appropriate recessive phenotypes resulting from a mitotic error, possibly a deletion, as a prerequisite for malignant transformation in a diploid cell.

This chapter is based on an analysis of the interchange between homologous mitotic chromosomes in the Bloom syndrome using the differential labeling method of sister chromatids with 5-bromodeoxyuridine (BrdU).[5,6] It suggests how chromatid exchanges may produce a cell which has become homozygous at many gene loci by somatic segregation.

MATERIALS AND METHODS

Cultured lymphocytes from 2 patients with the Bloom syndrome, 2 obligate heterozygotes, and 8 controls were exposed to 30 μg/ml 5-BrdU (Sigma, St. Louis) in the dark for 2 rounds of cell division and examined at metaphase as described elsewhere.[7] A total of 508 metaphases was studied (221 from patients, 120 from heterozygotes, and 167 from controls) under a fluorescence microscope after staining with 125 μg/ml acridine orange.[7]

RESULTS AND DISCUSSION

The sharp demarcation between one brightly fluorescent chromatid indicating the presence of one strand of original DNA, and one dull fluorescent chromatid (both DNA strands substituted with BrdU) was evident in the controls

*This investigation was supported in part by research grants from the Deutsche Forschungsgemeinschaft.

Birth Defects: Original Article Series, Volume XII, Number 1, pages 177–180

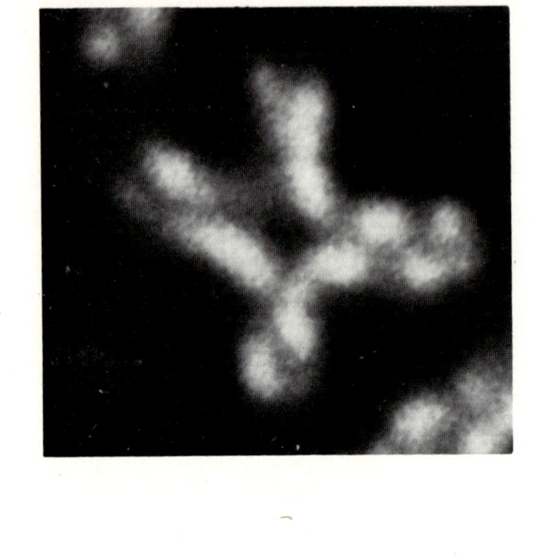

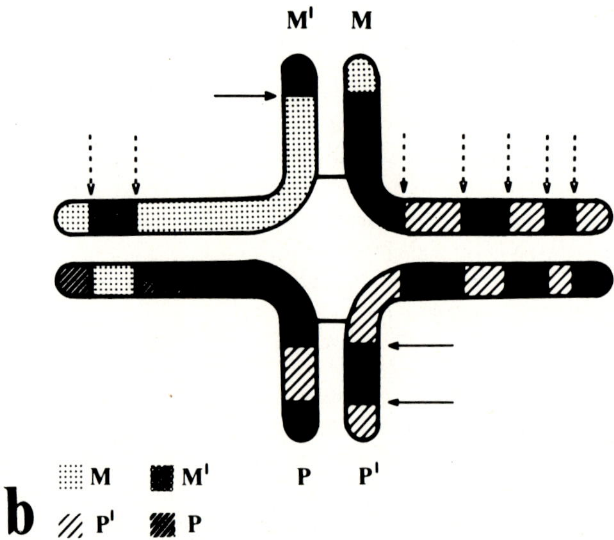

Fig. 1. A) Photograph and B) diagrammatic representation of chromatid exchanges involved in the formation of a quadriradial interchange figure at metaphase. Exchanges between sister chromatids are indicated by straight arrows, exchanges between homologous chromatids by arrows with broken line. The centromere is indicated by a thin line connecting the sister chromatids. M´ and P´ indicate the dull fluorescent newly replicated chromatids of maternal (M) and paternal (P) origin, respectively.

and the heterozygotes. The mean number of visible sister chromatid exchanges
(SCE) was 10.83 ± 3.58 (range 5.12–17.25) for the controls without age or
sex differences, and 10.45 ± 3.49 (range 4.5–20.5) for the heterozygotes.[7]
As reported recently,[8,9] the Bloom cells showed a striking increase in SCE
(90.58 ± 12.71, range 59.5–111).[7] In addition to the SCE, the occurrence
of homologous interchanges (Fig. 1A), although rare,[4,10] provides an opportunity for an exchange between chromatids of homologous chromosomes
(Fig. 1B). We suggest that this is a genetically important event, because recombinant chromosomes can result that have become homozygous at several
gene loci, if they were heterozygous before (Fig. 2). Consequently, recessive mutations can be expressed. Should somatic recombination of this type by chance
involve recessive genes which, in the homozygous state, are pertinent to malignant transformation, a monoclonal cell population differing from its host
could be established.

Patients with the Bloom syndrome have a predisposition to develop cancer in
tissues with high mitotic indices (bone marrow, lymphoid tissue, mucosal
cells of the gastrointestinal tract), a risk that apparently increases with age.[4]

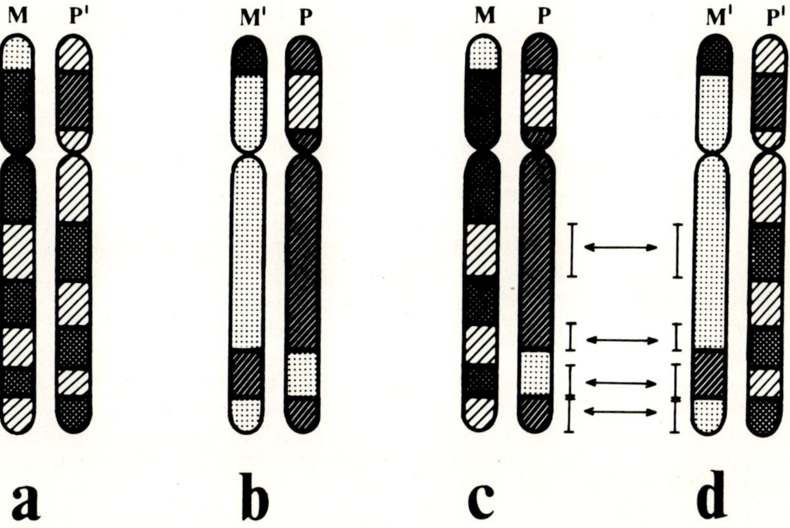

Fig. 2. Possible genetic consequences resulting from the chromatid exchanges shown
in Fig. 1. Following homologous chromatid exchanges recombinant chromosomes (c and d)
could be distributed to each of 2 daughter cells (in this case in the event of alternate segregation MP and M'P'). Genes located in the areas indicated by the 4 horizontal arrows
would have become homozygous by somatic recombination.

Obviously, opportunities for the formation of postzygotic homozygosity resulting from chromatid exchanges between homologous chromosomes are increased in such tissues.

Somatic segregation following chromatid exchanges between homologous chromosomes may thus be an important genetic consequence of the Bloom mutation in the homozygous state. We consider the possibility that this would favor the development of malignant cell clones.

This model is open to obvious criticism, because the rate of homologous exchanges is not increased in other disorders with chromosomal instability and predisposition to cancer. Nonetheless, what is very much amplified in the Bloom syndrome, could occasionally happen in other individuals as well. Chromatid exchanges between either homologous or nonhomologous chromosomes could occur in rapidly dividing tissues, and genes involved could be shifted from the heterozygous to the homozygous state. Somatic recombination and subsequent segregation could thus be envisioned as a source of cell populations capable of expressing recessive phenotypes.

REFERENCES

1. Burnet, Sir Macfarlane: The biology of cancer. In German, J. (ed.): "Chromosomes and Cancer," New York: John Wiley & Sons, 1974, pp. 21–38.
2. Whitehouse, H. L. K.: Chromosome integration of viral DNA: The open-replicon hypothesis of carcinogenesis. Ibid pp. 41–76.
3. Ohno, S.: Aneuploidy as a possible means employed by malignant cells to express recessive phenotypes. Ibid pp. 77–94.
4. German, J.: Bloom's syndrome. II. The prototype of human genetic disorders predisposing to chromosome instability and cancer. Ibid pp. 601–617.
5. Latt, S. A.: Microfluorometric detection of deoxyribonucleic acid replication in human metaphase chromosomes. Proc. Natl. Acad. Sci. USA 70:3395–3399, 1973.
6. Wolff, S. and Perry, P.: Differential Giemsa staining of sister chromatids and the study of sister chromatid exchanges without autoradiography. Chromosoma 48:341–353, 1974.
7. Bartram, C., Koske-Westphal, T. and Passarge, E.: Chromatid exchanges and somatic recombination in Bloom syndrome. Submitted for publication.
8. Chaganti, R. S. K., Schonberg, S. and German, J.: A manyfold increase in sister chromatid exchanges in Bloom's syndrome lymphocytes. Proc. Natl. Acad. Sci. USA 71: 4508–4512, 1974.
9. Sperling, K., Goll, U., Kunze, J. et al: Cytogenetic investigations in a new case of Bloom's syndrome. Submitted for publication.
10. Schroeder, T. M. and German, J.: Bloom's syndrome and Fanconi's anemia: Demonstration of two distinctive patterns of chromosome disruption and rearrangement. Humangenetik 25:299–306, 1974.

Noonan Syndrome - An Unusual Family with Above Average Intelligence, a High Incidence of Cancer and Rare Type of Vasculitis *

Martha S. Berberich, MD and Judith G. Hall, MD

Recently, we have seen a mother and daughter who have many features of classically described Noonan syndrome. However, they appear to differ from the usual Noonan syndrome patients because they are of normal height and above average intelligence. Other family members, who by history and pictures seemed to have physical features of the Noonan syndrome, were also of normal height and of above average to superior intelligence. Two of these adults died of vasculitis and 4 developed various cancers when they were over 35 years of age. We wish to raise the possibility that these disorders may be part of the natural history in some cases of Noonan syndrome. This family emphasizes the need for further studies to determine whether Noonan syndrome is a single syndrome with broad expressivity or a heterogeneous collection of disorders as yet not delineated.

CASE REPORTS

The proband (*VI-2*), (Fig. 1) a 5-year-old white female, was referred from the Cardiology Clinic because she had features of Noonan syndrome and a maternal history of congenital heart disease. Her weight and height were in the 3rd and 10th percentiles, respectively, for age. She had epicanthal folds, webbed neck, low posterior hairline, an increased carrying angle of her arms, and a moderate anterior chest deformity which was pectus carinatum superiorly and excavatum inferiorly (Fig. 2). On cardiac catheterization, mild-to-moderate valvular pulmonic stenosis was found.

Her mother, (*V-17*), had valvular pulmonic stenosis which had been corrected surgically. She was 5′6″ tall and had epicanthal folds, webbed neck, low posterior hairline, shield chest, pectus excavatum, increased carrying angle, and bilateral short 4th metacarpals (Fig. 3).

*Supported by NIH grants PO1 GM15253–08 and 5SO1 RR05655–07 and The National Foundation grants CA-90 and 6-75-174.

Birth Defects: Original Article Series, Volume XII, Number 1, pages 181–186
© 1976 The National Foundation

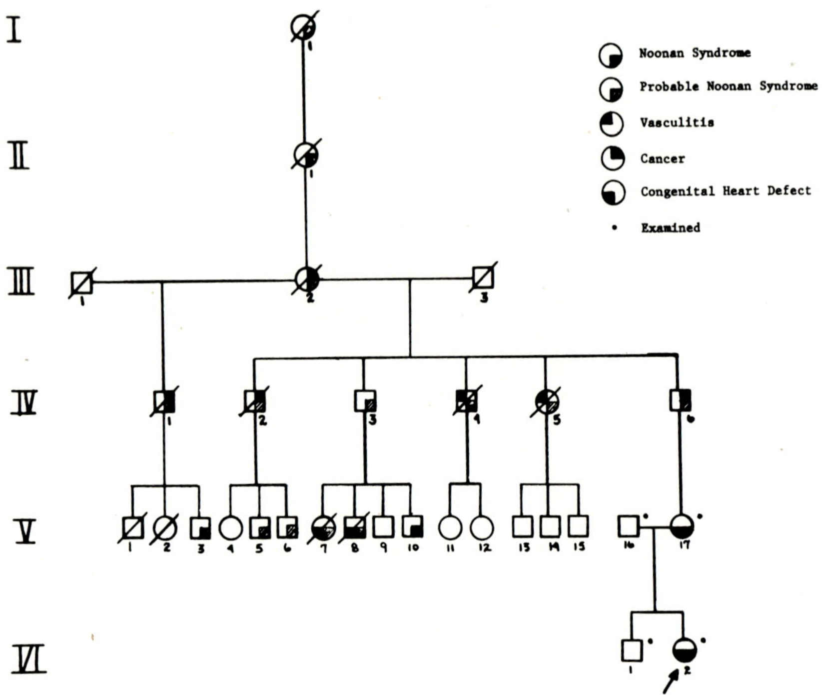

Fig. 1. Pedigree of family.

The brother and father of the proposita were examined. They were not affected.

Other family members were not examined because of death or residence in distant cities. The pedigree was constructed with the aid of family photographs and correspondence with several individuals, including the oldest living family member, who is a physician as well as the family historian.

From photographs (*I-1*), appears to have had ptosis, protuberant ears and a short, broad neck.

The great-grandmother, (*III-2*), of the proposita had kyphoscoliosis, a broad neck and low posterior hairline. She died in her 70s of bowel cancer.

The only child, (*IV-1*), by the first marriage of *III-2* was 5'10" tall. He had short stubby fingers with marked shortening of the 4th and 5th digits. He died at age 70 and the hospital diagnosis was cancer of the colon. His youngest son, (*V-3*), is 5'9" tall, has protuberant ears, a short neck, and low posterior hairline.

Another son, (*IV-2*) from a second marriage, was 5'8" tall. He had protuberant ears, malocclusion, and a slight pectus deformity. He died of biliary tract cancer. Two children, (*V-5* and *V-6*), have short necks and low posterior hairlines.

IV-3 is now 72 years old. Two of his children died of congenital heart disease in infancy. One had a patent ductus arteriosis, and the other a patent ductus

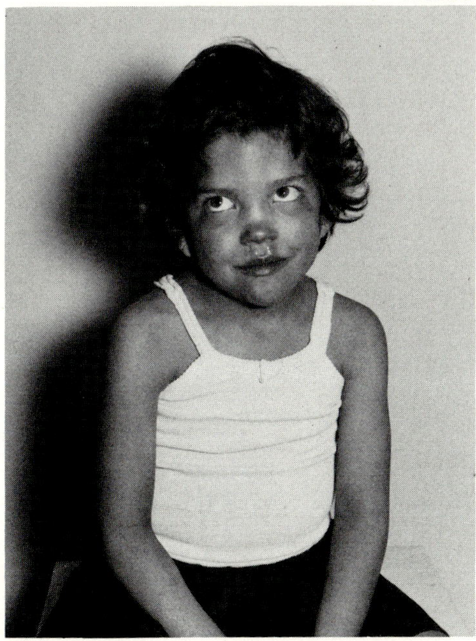

Fig. 2. Proposita (*VI-2*), age 5. Note epicanthal folds and webbed neck.

arteriosis and ventricular septal defect. His youngest child, (*V-10*), is 5′4″tall, has a short neck and short stubby fingers.

IV-4 was 5′10″ in height. He had protuberant ears, malocclusion, clinodactyly of both 5th fingers, and a pectus deformity. He died at age 68 and the autopsy diagnosis was Degos disease (malignant atrophic papulosis). The typical skin lesions, white depressed areas 2–3 mm in diameter with slightly erythematous margins, were present. In addition, vascular lesions were present but only in the intima of the vessels of the GI tract and CNS.

IV-5 was 5′5″ tall and had a low nuchal hairline. She died at age 48 with clinical and autopsy findings of polyserositis of unknown etiology. Chronic fibrinous pericarditis and subcapsular perisplenitis were present with vascular lupus erythematosus. The stomach and small intestine showed fibrinous areas on the serosa. For 3 years prior to her death, she had atrophic skin lesions and chronic weight loss. Family members, including a physician, noted the similarity of the skin lesions to those of her brother, (*IV-4*), when he became ill. The history and autopsy findings suggest that it is possible that she also had Degos disease.

The grandfather, (*IV-6*), of the proposita, is 5′11″ tall. He has a short neck, low nuchal hairline, and adult onset cataracts. He has biopsy-proven mycosis fungoides.

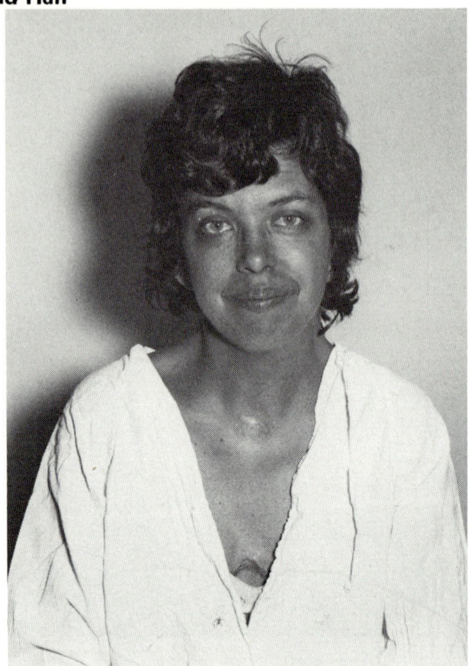

Fig. 3. Mother (*V-17*) of proposita. Note webbed neck.

DISCUSSION

This family is unusual in that the proposita and her mother have many of the classic features of Noonan syndrome, but are of normal stature and above average intelligence. Family members whom we believe to also have features compatible with Noonan syndrome include a former medical school dean, a state advisor for educational planning, 2 directors of self-owned construction firms, and an independent artist.

In this family, there appears to be an association between Noonan syndrome and cancer in later life. There have been 3 reported cases of Noonan syndrome associated with malignancy in children, but to our knowledge, no increased risk for malignancy at an older age in Noonan syndrome has been previously suggested. The tumors which have been reported in children were a ganglioneuroma,[1] a pheochromocytoma,[2] and a malignant schwannoma.[3] Interestingly, neural crest tumors accounted for 3 of 8 nongonadal malignancies reported in a series of Turner syndrome patients.[4] Although the family presented here is not a typical "cancer family" because the malignancies occurred late in life and the risk of malignancy in the general population is said to be 1 in 5,[5] the association seen in this family stresses the need for long-term follow-up of Noonan patients and their families to delineate the risk of developing cancer in patients with Noonan syndrome.

The occurrence of Degos disease in Noonan syndrome, or even in sibs has, to our knowledge, not been previously reported.[6] Since both are rare disorders, the association raises the possibility that some genetic abnormality in Noonan syndrome may predispose to the development of Degos disease. Degos disease has been reported in mother and son.[7] The etiology of Degos disease is unknown and, although an autoimmune basis has been suggested, there have been no consistent immunologic findings.[8,9] In this regard, it is of interest that patients with Noonan syndrome have been reported to have a high incidence of thyroiditis.[10] Since cardiomyopathy[11-13] has also been noted in some Noonan syndrome patients, it is possible that there is a generalized increased risk for autoimmune disorders in this syndrome. Alternatively, a molecular structural defect might account for the development of autoimmune and vascular disease and the late development of cancer.

As more cases are reported, there appears to be considerable heterogeneity in the Noonan syndrome and this family supports that impression. For example, the proposita and her mother demonstrate that normal height and normal intelligence can be seen in patients who otherwise have classic features of Noonan syndrome. We hope that this report stimulates interest in the further documentation of families with what is grouped, at the present time, under the name Noonan syndrome, so that more can be learned about its etiology, heterogeneity and natural history.

ACKNOWLEDGMENTS

The authors gratefully acknowledge referral of the family by Dr. Stanley Stamm and the technical assistance of Ellen Helseth.

REFERENCES

1. Khodadoust, A. and Paton, D.: Turner's syndrome in a male. Report of a case with myopia, retinal detachment, cataract and glaucoma. Arch. Ophthalmol. 77:630, 1967.
2. Becker, C. E., Rosen, S. W. and Engelman, K.: Pheochromocytoma and hyporesponsiveness to thyrotropin in a 46,XY male with features of Turner phenotype. Ann. Intern. Med. 70:325, 1969.
3. Kaplan, M. S., Opitz, J. M. and Grosset, F. R.: Noonan's syndrome. A case with elevated serum alkaline phosphatase levels and malignant schwannoma of the left forearm. Am. J. Dis. Child. 116:359, 1968.
4. Wertelecki, W., Fraumeni, J. F., Jr. and Mulvihill, J. J.: Nongonadal neoplasia in Turner's syndrome. Cancer 26:485, 1970.
5. Stevenson, A. C., Davison, B. C. C. and Oakes, M. W.: Neoplasms. In "Genetic Counseling." Philadelphia: J. B. Lippincott, Co., 1970, p. 283.

6. Strole, W. E., Clark, W. H., Jr. and Isselbacher, K. J.: Progressive arterial occlusive disease (Kohlmeier-Degos). A frequently fatal cutaneosystemic disorder. N. Engl. J. Med. 276:195, 1967.

7. Hall-Smith, P.: Malignant atrophic papulosis (Degos' disease). Two cases occurring in the same family. Br. J. Derm. 81:817, 1969.

8. Roenigk, H. H. and Farmer, R. G.: Degos' disease (malignant papulosis). Report of three cases with clues to etiology. JAMA 206:1508, 1968.

9. Black, M. M., Nichioka, K. and Levene, G. M.: The role of dermal blood vessels in the pathogenesis of malignant atrophic papulosis (Degos' disease). Br. J. Derm. 88:213, 1973.

10. Vesterhus, P. and Aarskog, D.: Noonan syndrome and autoimmune thyroiditis. J. Pediatr. 83:237, 1973.

11. Phornphutkel, C., Rosenthal, A. and Nadas, A. S.: Cardiomyopathy in Noonan syndrome. Report of three cases. Br. Heart J. 35:99, 1973.

12. Williams, G. H., Rose, L. I., Jagger, P. I. and Lauler, D. P.: A Turner's syndrome variant with polycystic ovaries and idiopathic myocardial hypertrophy. Ann. Intern. Med. 70:571, 1969.

13. Bolton, M. R., Pugh, D. M., Mattiolo, L. F. et al: The Noonan syndrome. A family study. Ann. Intern. Med. 80:626, 1974.

Trisomy 8 Mosaicism in the Skin of a Patient with Leukemia

Vincent M. Riccardi, MD

We have recently evaluated a family with a heritable, balanced reciprocal translocation [t(7p;20p)] spanning at least 3 generations. The proband was a 42-year-old white male with acute granulocytic leukemia (AGL). The translocation was discovered in the work-up of his leukemia, and has been demonstrated in T lymphocytes, skin fibroblasts and AGL blast cells of the bone marrow. In addition, he showed mosaic trisomy 8 (T8) in his marrow blasts (about 20%) and skin fibroblasts (13%). Although mosaic T8 has been demonstrated in the malignant cells of AGL and other hematologic malignancies,[1] it has not been shown to be concurrently present in skin fibroblasts. The precise relationship of the 2 chromosome aberrations to each other and to the AGL is not clear, although it would seem from these data that the T8 was neither a coincidental marker nor a consequence of the leukemia. Additional investigations are underway to establish the association of the heritable translocation with the 4 additional maternal relatives who have developed malignancies (1 leukemia and 3 carcinomas).[2]

In any case, the importance of this preliminary report is to emphasize the need to study the skin fibroblast chromosomes in other patients with hematologic malignancies. Before conclusions are drawn about the significance of the extra chromosome in leukemia cells its presence in other tissues of the patient must be clarified.

REFERENCES

1. Hsu, L. Y. F., Alter, A. V. and Hirschhorn, K.: Trisomy 8 in bone marrow cells of polycythemia vera and myelogenous leukemia. Clin. Genet. 6:258–264, 1974.
2. Riccardi, V. M., Humbert, J. and Peakman, D.: Familial cancer, reciprocal translocation [t(7p;20p)] and trisomy 8. Abstract submitted for presentation to the American Society of Human Genetics, Baltimore, MD, October, 1975.

Selected Abstracts

MUCOSAL NEUROMA SYNDROME WITH MEDULLARY THYROID CARCINOMA — REPORT OF CASE

Penny A. Bard, Leslie A. Bard and Charles E. Kesmodel

Departments of Pediatrics and Ophthalmology, Kaiser Foundation Hospital, Sacramento, California

A 13 7/12-year-old caucasian boy was found to have typical features of the mucosal neuroma syndrome (MNS) on ophthalmoligic examination. The paternal family history was markedly suggestive of multiple endocrine neoplasia (MEN) Type II. He was immediately referred to his pediatrician for evaluation of possible medullary thyroid carcinoma (MCT) and pheochromocytoma (PCC).

The patient had neuromas of the tongue, lips, and penis; a history of meatotomy for structure at age 8 years, and a lifelong history of obstipation. There was a congenital talipes equinovarus on the left with recurrence after each of 3 operations. A marfanoid habitus was evident with progressive loss of subcutaneous fat and muscle wasting. Dry eyes since age 2 years required therapy with artificial tears. Neuromas of the lids and conjunctiva appeared in early childhood, and the diagnosis was established by the pathognomonic slit-lamp appearance of thickened corneal nerves which had been present since at least age 9 years. Once the diagnosis was made, palpation of the neck revealed 3 nodules in the area of the thyroid gland. This led to his hospital admission in February, 1975.

Multiple blood pressure measurements had been normal over the previous 6 years and remained so. All blood, serum, and urine tests were normal except slight elevation of the PM serum cortisol and a markedly elevated unstimulated serum calcitonin on 2 separate days. Twenty-four hour urinary

Birth Defects: Original Article Series, Volume XII, Number 1, pages 189—194

VMA excretion was normal. Skull and chest x-ray films were normal. Metacarpal index (8.8) was above upper range of normal. Bone age (hand) was 2½ years retarded at age 11 years and preoperatively. Thyroid scan (Tc99) showed diffusely decreased uptake; none of the 3 nodules showed any activity. IVP was normal and barium enema showed a normal colon.

Operation consisted of total thyroidectomy and radical neck dissection. One normal parathyroid gland was removed. Five lymph nodes with metastatic MCT were found, and the thyroid was dissected from the trachea with difficulty, suggesting inoperable local infiltration. Pathologic examination showed a typical MCT with amyloid deposit. Postoperative course was uneventful.

Since most patients so far reported with MEN Type II and MNS have had metastatic disease from MCT, we want to emphasize the importance of early recognition. Recent reports have documented that both MCT and PCC car. be diagnosed in the premalignant hyperplasia stage. Early surgery will hopefully prevent much of the morbidity and mortality of this disease.

THE VON RECKLINGHAUSEN SYNDROME

Stella B. Kontras

Department of Pediatrics, College of Medicine, Ohio State University, Children's Hospital, Columbus, Ohio

Fifty-five children with neurofibromatosis have been studied at Columbus Children's Hospital from 1952 to 1975. As suggested by Feinman (1970), criteria used for the diagnoses were 5 or more café-au-lait spots greater than 0.5 cm in diameter, positive family history or biopsy proven neurofibromas. In that series, a 15% incidence of tumors was reported, primarily intracranial in location. In our series of children, only 3 have been found to have tumors. These were not intracranial but included a thoracic ganglioneuroma, an ovarian teratoma and a soft tissue sarcoma (incidence of 4%). A further pedigree on one of these families is of interest in that 4 affected generations are present (11 patients affected). The index case, an 8-year-old boy, was referred for scalp tumors and was noted to have numerous café-au-lait spots and neurofibromatosis. His mother died of meningioma at age 40 but had produced 8 children by 5 matings, all of whom are affected, except a 2 year old. This group of sibs demonstrates many described complications of the von Recklinghausen syndrome including skin lesions, tumors, mental retardation, growth failure, renal hypertension, hypoglycemia, glaucoma and seizures. The mother's mother, who was affected, died of carcinomatosis (breast carcinoma) and her mother, also affected, died of cancer (type unknown).

This family illustrates the need for clinical recognition of the von Recklinghausen disease for genetic counseling to the affected individuals, and for knowledge of and surveillance for the complications, including tumors.

MULTIPLE MUCOSAL NEUROMA SYNDROME

Jules G. Leroy

Laboratory of Genetics and Medical Genetics, Antwerp University, Antwerp, Belgium

Proband is the 21-year-old second boy in a family of four. His unrelated healthy parents were 26 and 25 years at the time he was born. Two brothers and one sister, the youngest sib, are also normal. Frequent bouts of GI problems, intermittent infectious skin lesions and rather slow psychomotor development were the main parental complaints during his infancy and early childhood. Thick blubbery lips were already mentioned at that time, when pink nodules were also noticed on the anterior dorsal surface of the tongue. At age 7, he underwent orthopedic surgery for bilateral pes cavus. Episodes of asthmatic respiratory difficulties, first apparent about the age of 9 years, have improved considerably. At 16 years, following a period of painful walking, he had a slipped upper femoral epiphysis on the right side, requiring 2 surgical interventions. Two years ago, some nodules were removed from the margin of the right lower eyelid.

The patient was first seen in 1974 and the diagnosis of multiple mucosal neuroma syndrome was made. He was 181 cm tall and had a slightly Marfanoid general appearance. He had several small pink tumors on the anterior dorsal surface of the tongue and similar lesions seated more deeply in the buccal mucosa and in both lips. Identical tumors were detected on the vocal cords. Microscopic inspection revealed thickened nerve fibers anastomosing within the pupillary region of the corneal stroma. Except for a stiff right hip, the patient has increased mobility of all large and small joints. He wears orthopedic shoes because of both the persisting pes cavus and the unequal length of the lower limbs.

Radiographic studies revealed a postoperative status of the right hip, dolichomegacolon and megaloureter. Routine laboratory tests have yielded normal results. Thyroid function appeared normal. A thyroid scan did not show abnormalities. There was no clinical evidence of pheochromocytoma, and urinary catecholamines were normal. The amount of plasma calcitonin however, was found to be more than 30 times the control values. Biopsy specimens of the tongue lesions and of the thyroid gland are currently being studied. This patient is an isolated case in the family pedigree. His disease is probably due to a new mutation in the germinal cells in one of his parents.

CHROMOSOME CHANGES ASSOCIATED WITH THE LOSS OF MALIGNANT CHARACTERISTICS IN A HUMAN MENINGIOMA

Ian H. Porter and Betty Paul

Birth Defects Institute, New York State Department of Health, Albany, New York

Cells from most meningiomas are *hypo*diploid with a consistent loss of a G-22 chromosome. This loss has been implicated as the initial phase in the development of cytogenetic abnormalities of this tumor.

We have established a subline from a cultured meningioma that originally contained chromosomal modes of 38 and 39, chromosomes missing from groups A, C, D, E and G, and a long acrocentric marker chromosome in 100% of the cells.

Our subline contains a *hyper*diploid mode of 66 chromosomes and a long acrocentric marker chromosome in 100% of the cells. Additional chromosomes are present in the groups affected by chromosome loss in the original tumor.

Morphologically these cells resemble a normal (nontransformed) cultured line, are contact inhibited, do not form colonies in soft agar, and tumors are not produced when 10^6 and 1.5×10^6 cells are injected subcutaneously in 3-day-old immunosuppressed Swiss mice. The gain of a G-22 chromosome and the suppression of the malignant state may be related, and we may thus be able to examine the chromosomal involvement in the malignant process by examining revertants of this line.

ATAXIA-TELANGIECTASIA — AN IN VITRO MARKER

P. Sargent, R. Finkelberg and D. I. Hoar

Department of Medical Genetics, University of Toronto, Toronto, Ontario, Canada

Ataxia-telangiectasia (A-T) has been grouped with the chromosomal breakage syndromes which show an increased tendency towards malignancy. Recently, in vitro markers have been identified in fibroblasts from patients with Fanconi anemia (FA) and Bloom syndrome (BS). FA cells show enhanced mitomycin-C sensitivity; BS lymphocytes show increased sister chromatid exchanges. No marker has yet been reported for A-T fibroblasts.

In conducting a survey of cell lines for sensitivity to chemical agents, we chose to examine actinomycin-D sensitivity, since this agent is known to stimulate centromere region recombination in drosophila. Dose-response survival curves with actinomycin-D revealed that A-T skin-derived fibroblasts have an enhanced sensitivity. The results of screening with actinomycin-D and several other chemical agents on A-T and FA cells will be discussed.

MOUSE LYMPHOMA AS AN EXPERIMENTAL MODEL FOR HUMAN NEOPLASIA

F. Sergovich, F. Chan, J. Ball and M. Smout

The Children's Psychiatric Research Institute, The Cancer Research Laboratory, University of Western Ontario and Department of Pathology, Victoria Hospital, London, Canada

Salient features of ataxia-telangiectasia include the finding of chromosome breaks in cultured cells, and a predisposition to malignancy of the lymphoreticular system. There are increasing numbers of reports showing that patients in vivo preferentially accumulate a clone of cells in which a highly specific chromosome abnormality exists, and it has been interesting to speculate that this was related to, or perhaps been indicative of, premalignant change. However, experimental manipulation of patients is limited by ethical considerations and the rarity of the disorder. Our preliminary data indicate that this hurdle can be overcome using Mus musculus.

Fifty newborn mice (CFW/D strain) were injected with 7, 12 DMBA; 15 of these died within 2 weeks. Twenty surviving mice showed evidence of tumor at latent periods varying from 70 to 183 days and these were sacrificed for chromosome studies. Nine of these mice had a thymus of normal size and few mitotic figures. One died immediately after colcemide injection. The remaining 19 form the core of the study.

The chromosome complements in 18 of these were not always identical but they generally fell into 2 groups when analyzed with quinacrine fluorescence and direct flame-dry techniques: those which were solely trisomic for chromosome 15, and those which were trisomic for chromosome 15 but contained an additional anomaly — usually another trisomy but some had "marker" chromosomes. Only one tumor was chromosomally normal. This experiement was repeated using the C57/B1 strain. In this instance the incidence of tumors with a normal chromosome complement was greatly increased (8 of 26) indicating a strong strain response to carcinogen. Nonetheless, trisomy 15 was characteristically found in at least 50% of the cells in the remaining 18, although in a variety of combinations with different cytogenetic anomalies.

These preliminary data strongly suggest that chemical carcinogenesis in the mouse is a useful experimental model for the study of the premalignant and neoplastic processes in man.

EFFECT OF VINCRISTINE ON CHROMOSOMES

Claude Stoll, Digamber S. Borgaonkar and Jean-Marc Levy

Division of Medical Genetics, Department of Medicine, The Johns Hopkins University School of Medicine, Baltimore, Maryland and Clinique Infantile, Hôpital Civil, Strasbourg, France

Analysis of human lymphocyte cultures treated with BrdU and acridine orange after addition of vincristine demonstrates that it has an inhibitory effect on chromosomes. The dosage-effect of vincristine is demonstrated when it is added to cultures during the first 24 hours. Second mitosis does not progress, and if it does, the sister chromatid exchanges are decreased when compared to controls.

Author Index

Subject Index

A

ACTH, 35
Adenocarcinomas, follicular, 7
Adenomas
    fetal, 7
    pituitary (chromophobic), 94
    sebaceous, 9
Adenomatosis, 103
Adenosine deaminase, 66
Adenosquamous carcinoma, 29
Adenovirus, 12, 114
Age
    distribution of cancer, 1
    lung cancer, 100
Agonadia, 42
Allografts, 72
Alpha$_1$-antitrypsin deficiency, 8, 105
Alveolar cell carcinoma, 101, 106
Amenorrhea, 31, 40
American Indians, lung cancer, 99
Amethopterin, 115
Androgen, 32
Aneuploidy, 31, 80
Angioma, 93
Angioreticuloma, 93
Angiolipomas, cutaneous, 10
Aniridia, 4
Anorchia, 42
Antibodies, tumor-specific, 62
Antibody-secreting cells, 63
Antigens
    cell-surface, 31
    tumor-specific transplantation, 61
    virus-induced tumors, 61
Aplasia, femoral, 173
Arrhenoblastomas, 56
Aryl hydrocarbon hydroxylase, 104
Ashkenazi Jews, 141
Astrocytomas, 93, 94
Ataxia-telangiectasia, 68, 115, 116, 135, 192
Autosomal dominant traits, 103

Autosomal recessive traits, 115
    lung cancer, 104, 106
    syndromes, 133, 134*

B

Banding techniques, 114
β-cell system, defects, 66
β lymphocytes, 63
Blacks
    Ewing tumor, 2
    lung cancer, 99
    tumors, 53
Bladder cancer, 102
Blood group B, 105
Bloom syndrome, 115, 116, 141, 177
Blue rubber bleb nevus, 9
Bone marrow, 117
Breast cancer, 3, 7, 32, 101
    families, 156
    heredity, 141
    hermaphrodites, 34
Brenner tumors, 24
Bronchogenic carcinoma, 100
Burkitt lymphoma, 62, 117, 127–129
    clones, 124
Bursa of Fabricius, 63

C

Café-au-lait spots, 133
Calcitonin, 159
Calcium tests, 159
Cancer family syndrome, 151
Candida albicans, 68
Carcinoid, 106
Central nervous system
    developmental errors, 95
    tumors, 94, *95*
Cervical cancer, 102
Chediak-Higashi syndrome, 141
Chemodectomas, 8
Chlorodinitrobenzene, 62
Children, cancer, 2

*Italicized numbers refer to tables.